FAMILY PRESCRIPTION

FAMILY PRESCRIPTION

A HISTORY OF A FAMILY

WENDY ELMQUIST

Tate Publishing & *Enterprises*

Published by Tate Publishing & Enterprises, LLC
127 E. Trade Center Terrace | Mustang, Oklahoma 73064 USA
1.888.361.9473 | www.tatepublishing.com

Tate Publishing is committed to excellence in the publishing industry. The company reflects the philosophy established by the founders, based on Psalm 68:11,
"The Lord gave the word and great was the company of those who published it."

Cover design by Kellie Southerland
Interior design by Jeff Fisher
Author photo courtesy Jaderborg Photography, Tom Jaderborg, Lindsborg, KS.
Thank You: Alycia Banks, Stylist, Peabody, KS.

Published in the United States of America

ISBN: 978-1-61566-463-4
1. Self-Help, Substance Abuse & Addictions, Drug Dependence
2. Family & Relationships, General
10.02.09

DEDICATION

To my parents: Thank you for picking me.

To my husband, Dean: I'm glad I picked you. Thank you for being my best friend, for loving me, and for never giving up on me. You taught me what love is and how to love.

To my girls, Jennifer and Angie, who were always there through thick and thin and to your families. I love you all.

To Gary, my brother: I'm glad you got picked and you became my brother, and to you and your family, thanks for your support and for the laughter.

To the rest of the family and friends along the way: Thanks for everything.

A special thanks to my dad for believing in me and always loving me.

—Love, Wendy

P.S. To my three angels, I know you're there.

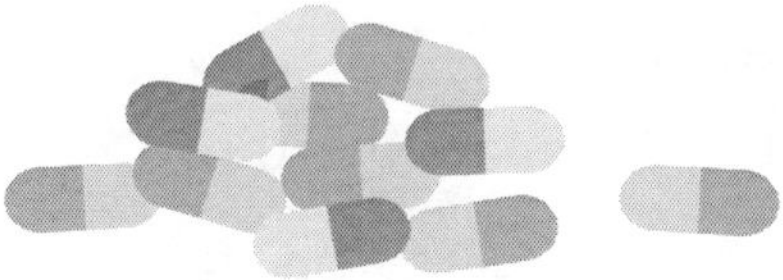

TABLE OF CONTENTS

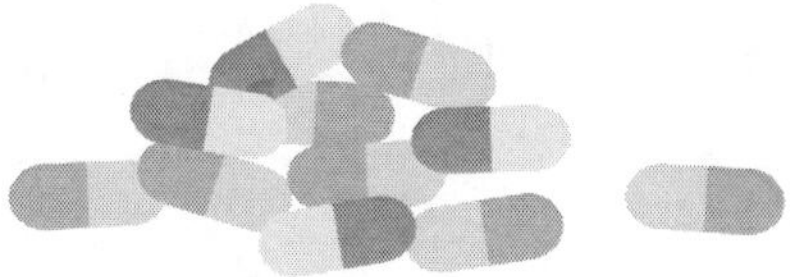

WELCOME TO THE FAMILY PRESCRIPTION

Have you ever taken someone else's prescription medicine before?

Have you ever given a friend or relative your prescription medicine?

What would you do if you caught your child or your child's friend taking prescription medication out of your purse? Or even worse, taking either your medication or over the counter (OTC) out of your medicine cabinet?

What if you received a call, saying that your child or possibly your parent had been taken to the ER because he or she had taken the wrong medicine or accidentally overdosed and was unconscious or was pronounced dead?

Or a possibility of missed diagnosed and almost paying with your health or with your life?

Do I Have Your Attention Now?

My name is Wendy, and this is my story about prescription drugs. With the strength of my family, and God, I'm still here. This story could have happened to anyone, but it happened to me, and I hope or wish that anyone who reads my story can help a child, teenager, or any adult. My intent is to tell the facts of how prescription drugs and their effects can change a life.

I absolutely hate illegal drugs and what they do to a body, but taking the wrong prescription medicine can have the same effect. Illegal, legal, or over-the-counter drugs can do damage and cause a loss in life. I want to tell about my journey through withdrawal hell and what can happen to your body and soul. If you live through withdrawal, the after effects can stay with you the rest of your life. This is why I named my story *Family Prescription.* Life can be like a game of chess, and your next move might be your last. Your family will try to protect you and guard you against these forces. I want to take you back in the past and present how I was raised up on a farm by Lindsborg, Kansas.

Lindsborg, Kansas

Little Sweden, USA

The Town–Välkommen–Welcome

Upon entering the town of around 3,000, you will notice the brick lined streets and hear the Swedish music. As you are walking around shopping, this might put a jig in your step. The stores are painted with each owners taste and the window shopping doesn't even begin to show you the merchandise that has been imported from Sweden. Each store has it's own inventory, so there is something new and different around every corner.

This town is very lucky to be able to have it's needs looked after. Small towns depend on the bigger cities for help.

Education

The educational needs for the Smoky Valley area, which includes pre-K through 12th grades. A four year, liberal arts college, sits in the town area. Bethany College prides itself on the dedication of professors and is in the KCAC Conference.

Health

The medical facilities and medical staff work around the clock. The doctor's offices, Pharmacy, (Apotek) and the Lindsborg Community Hospital, are all in one area. When you are being treated, you notice you are a person and not a number.

The volunteers of Lindsborg are really something. Both our fire and ambulance departments are on twenty-four hour call and do a fantastic job. If an emergency should arise, you will be shipped out either by ambulance or helicopter.

Our elderly care is provided by Bethany Home. The residences are treated with the utmost care and dignity. All their needs are met. Their schedule keeps them hopping and one of the favorite activities is the trolley car. The trolley is great on the beautiful days in Kansas. Lots of fresh air and even a wave is just the prescription.

To spend a night or two, you have lots of options to choose from. There are several lovely bed and breakfasts and two hotels, which are independently run.

There is one inn our family has worked for, sharing many wonderful times seeing to the needs of our guests. The innkeepers of the Swedish Country Inn work tirelessly around the clock to meet all their guests needs, with the Swedish heritage and the way they were brought up in Lindsborg. They strive to show the Swedish ambience in everything they do. The best part is waking to the smell of coffee and a Swedish breakfast buffet.

You will have no problem finding a wonderful meal. American, Swedish, and Mexican, are just a few ideas. The bakeries always have the coffee on with wonderful pastries and maybe you would like to try a Swedish pancake. I want to give you a hint–the coffee pot better, never go dry in Lindsborg.

When your bones are weary from sight seeing and you would enjoy a great sandwich, Ol Stuga is the place to go. Mark makes the best sandwiches and you can have a cold beer with your meal.

There is one grocery store, that goes out of its way to provide the usual choice in food, but the Swedish cuisine, they import a lot of items from the Scandinavian region. Scott's prepares a lot of Swedish food items for the surrounding area. Fresh Swedish rye bread is a favorite, potato sausage, Swedish meatball mix and a favorite Swedish dessert, ostkaka.

They import from Sweden other foods such as lingonberries, cheese's and lutefisk.

What is lutefisk?

It's not my favorite but it's a fish from Sweden and come fresh, frozen, or dried. You can fix it different ways, but creaming it seems to be the best. My grandparents and my brother Gary, liked it and always had a dinner together, after the Christmas holidays. Gary's breathe always smelled real bad when he came home but seemed to enjoy proving it to me. I often have wondered what is does to your digestive system, when after a meal, you have to re-polish the silverware because there is something about lutefisk.

Religion

On Sunday mornings you are greeted with the ringing of the church bells, welcoming you to services. There are several denominations in Lindsborg. Each one would enjoy having you participate in the service. But there is one church that holds so many events in my life. Bethany Lutheran Church has been my family's base for many years. When my girls were both confirmed, they represented the fifth generation from our family tree.

But from far away, you can see the white steeple, with the large trees protecting it, this has become an icon, to me.

Castle on the Hill

I always know when I'm close to home, when I catch site of a hill that is standing watch over the Smokey Valley area. Coronado Heights is a wonderful place to go and look the country side over. There is a rock castle on the very top, that you can stand on the very top and see the surrounding area. Sometimes, the fields look like a beautiful patchwork quilt. The castle and the road that wraps around the hill, was built by the Workers Progress Administration, (WPA). My family used to enjoy taking a picnic basket up when it was hot, but it always seemed cooler up there. Dad would always stop half way up and let us off so we could run up the stairs, built on the side of the hill. We would try to see who got to the top, first. Sometimes dad would let us win.

When visiting Lindsborg, there are many events, taking place around the calendar. There is something for everyone.

The Heritage of Lindsborg

One of the main events will be happening this year, the second weekend in October. The Svensk Hyllingsfest is a great weekend to visit with friends and family. The traveler that come from far and wide enjoy being involved in the Swedish heritage.

Events include the crowning of the king and queen, craft tents set up around town and lots of Swedish dancing in the streets. Friday night, if you can buy a ticket to one of the three settings, a Swedish Smorgasbord is served on the college campus and I would say don't eat much during the day, save room. On Saturday, the day begins with the annual parade following with another presentation of Fridays events and even more programs are scheduled. In the afternoon, the homecoming football game is played, which is a lot of fun.

When Sunday rolls around and after the days events are done and everyone has gone home, when the sun is setting, you can hear Lindsborg take in a big breathe. She knows a good time was had by all and another Hyllinngsfest is in the history books.

Palm and Easter Sunday's

Every year Handel's "Messiah" is performed by the residents of the Smoky Valley area with the help from the students of Bethany College. All through Holy week, are concerts by the soloists. My favorite happens on Good Friday. Bach, (St. Matthews Passion) is my favorite performance and it's a wonderful way to spend a religious holiday.

Other yearly events are Mills Fest and, in June, Midsommardag (Midsummer's Day).

This event is held in the park where the Swedes celebrate the longest day of the year. First, the Swedish National Anthem, is sung, and the day is long. Of course with craft booths and Swedish dancing and programs, food booths where you might even get a bowl of homemade ice cream. There are booths just for the kids, where they learn how to make something Swedish. This event is being held in our sister city, Munkfor's Sweden. In the evening, the day is closed in the Old Mill Park, where the Swedish dancers, dance the popular May Pole. If you sit towards the front, you might be asked to dance with one of the dancers. This is a nice way to end a very long day…

The Christmas Holidays

This is my favorite time, when Lindsborg is lit up all over. Between Thanksgiving and Christmas Eve, every weekend there is something happening. From the lighting of the lights on the iron bridge, the snowflake- tomte parade, celebrating St. Lucia and all those special nights of shopping and enjoying treats in the stores. Some of the residents have an open house, to see how they decorate their homes. But the best part, on the last two weekends before Christmas is spending the evening at the Old Mill. It's the old fashion Christmas, like it was in the pioneer days of the 1880s. Walking through the gate and hearing the carolers, walking the planked walks and stopping to talk to the pioneers about how they were spending the holidays. If you are lucky, there might be a few snowflakes lightly flowing through the air. If you don't have the Christmas spirit. When you walk away, you will feel it.

On Christmas morning, in celebrating the birth of the Baby Jesus, a service is held at Bethany Church at 6am. There is beautiful stained-glass window and behind them a glow that makes them stand out, a little more.

You enter the church and you realize where the glow is coming from. The service is a candle light service and called Julotta. My father, in his teenage years, was one who played his trombone up in the bell tower. He also comments on how cold it was.

My uncle Ernie once commented on how the Swedes have a strange time to celebrate a birthday. I looked over at my grandfather, as he lowered his chin, with a sheepish grin.

Main Street is a beautiful sight when the snow is light and the white lights show off all the Swedish colors from the buildings. It will take your breathe away.

The reason I put Lindsborg first is because, the town of Lindsborg is a very important part of the prescription and starts the History of a Family…

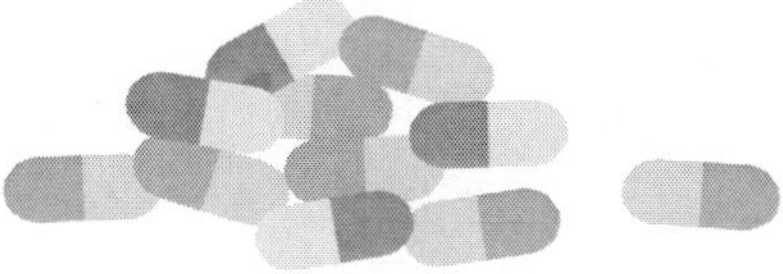

MY DAD

My dad's name is Leroy Andrew Sundberg and if I had to describe him I would say. He is the most honest, hard-working man. He was also the man who loved my mother very much and still to this day, takes care of us. He is the man that if you fell off the horse, he would put you back on, and he taught us how to respect, love had greet what life gives you, and is still showing us how to keep the faith and the power of strength. He is also the man that called me "Tootsie" and to this day, I still melt.

Born January 1921, he was the eldest son of Fred and Ethel Sundberg. Dad lived most of his years on the farm near Lindsborg.

The house at the time of his birth was built in 1914. Dad's grandfather, Andrew Daniel, gave a carpenter in Lindsborg, 1,325 dollars to build a two-story, four-bedroom farmhouse. In the downstairs den is where Dad and his three other siblings were given life.

The house took two long years to finish since the carpenter worked by himself and never hired any help. When Andrew Daniel decided to retire and move to town, Fred and Ethel took over the family farm. When my grandfather decided to retire and move to town, Dad, being the oldest, took over the farm, so it has been passed down through many generations. This was what was expected of you during those times. When Dad and Mom moved to town in 1979, they rented the house and ten acres to several different people until Dad couldn't take care of it, and it was sold.

Being brought up on the farm, my grandfather was a good farmer, and Dad learned from his father how to take care of his family, and at that time farming wasn't a booming business. Dad tells the story of how they used to work the fields with horse-drawn farm equipment. One day while mowing with his father—Dad was around eight or nine years old—he was helping change the sickle because the blade had become dull, and he lost a finger. My father never took any chances with us about riding on the farm equipment and this is probably why.

When going to church, they drove their Model A to town for services and Luther League, which was for the youth. He was baptized and confirmed by Dr. Alfred Bergin, who accepted the call to succeed the late Dr. Carl Swenson to Bethany Lutheran Church in 1904 in which the town and church were established in 1869.

Dad and his brothers and sister went to Fallquist School. A short walk from home was a one-room school in which they had a teacher who taught grades one through eight and had a total of nine students. Dad went to high school in Lindsborg. Lindsborg High School was where Grandpa, Dad, Gary, and I, plus my husband, Dean, and our daughters received our diplomas.

Dad was always very busy on the farm, but I asked him one day if he had a hobby he enjoyed doing. He replied reading books and studying by kerosene lamp. They didn't have electricity yet, but they had a radio, but their bedtimes came early due to the chores they were expected to have done before school.

Dad said that in the dust bowl days, the heat was tremendous, and they would have to go in out of the heat and lay on the linoleum floors in order to keep cool. No air conditioning or carpeting was in the homes during this time. I remember Grandma telling the story about when the grasshoppers exploded onto the scene, and the chickens would eat so many hoppers that their eggs tasted so different and using them became difficult. Dad told me that the neighbor's pet turkeys would manage to eat their way to their house, and they would have to chase them home.

The Depression came, but they really didn't feel the blast like the larger towns did. They had everything they needed to survive on the farm: milk from the cows and eggs and meat from the chickens. They butchered their own beef and pork. They would go hunting or fishing if they wanted something different to eat. Their huge garden and the fruit trees in the orchard, when grandma canned, was enough to get through the year. Grandpa was a believer in potatoes at least once a day, so he worked on a huge plot of ground where he planted the potatoes, and they would keep them in the basement where the canned items were also kept. He thought that was a good way to keep his boys' stomachs full.

In July of '42, Dad enlisted in the United States Navy Reserves, active duty because the next day his number in the lottery was coming up, so between Salina and Kansas City is where he took his preliminaries and became a naval air cadet. Then he was ordered to Wichita University for ground school, and at the Wichita Airport was taught in a small plane to fly and transferred in '43 to Monterey, California andfor three more months of preflight and ground school and on to Norman, Oklahoma. At this small naval base was where he learned to fly a bi-wing with an open cockpit.

After four months he was ordered to Corpus Christi, Texas, where he completed and graduated from flight training and received his naval wings. This was a very proud day in his life. He went on and received his plane commander commission, which sent him to Oakland, California, where he received his crew and flew a four engine R5D. This is where my mom entered the picture, but two or three weeks later, he was ordered to Honolulu where he would fly a route from Oakland to Honolulu and Guam. He didn't get to see Mom but every three to four weeks but usually had a week off until he was called back to duty. His crew was responsible for freight and supplies and naval personnel to their next bases where they were ordered to go. A lot of the flights were for the beginning of the Korean conflict. Dad and his crew were also responsible for bringing wounded personnel home at the end of the war from Japan. In 1946, his orders took him back to Oakland where he and Mom were married. They had dated on and off for a year. He was stationed at Moffet Field, and soon after their marriage, they continued onto Dad's next assignment in Seattle, Washington, where he would fly to Adak, Atka, Nome, Anchorage, and Kodiak, where he was transferred back to base in Seattle on orders from his close friend, George Tubbs, because dad had become a new father.

This is where I am ending his story because the upcoming chapters will explain his next steps.

MY MOM

My mom's maiden name was Doris June Swanson. She hated her middle name, and she made us promise not to put it on her headstone. She was the first and only daughter of Oscar and Flo Swanson. She was born in March of 1927. She and her brother Donald (Duke) had a very close relationship. Their parents each worked, so they spent a lot of time by themselves.

Duke took over as mom's bodyguard. He used to say, "Someone had to watch over her." He did his job very well, although he was fifteen months younger and built smaller. But he was a pretty scrappy little guy.

They always looked forward to Saturdays and Sundays. They went downtown, and if Grandpa won at poker, they would go to the show and ice cream. They always saw the show and got ice cream after. Grandpa was an excellent poker player, and Duke is still a good poker player. He was taught well.

Sometimes Grandpa would even provide for their friends. Mom's parents were one of the lucky ones through the Depression. They had good jobs, and I'm sure they felt the Depression in California, but Mom said that Grandma used to make sure it didn't enter their house.

Mom's father never liked the idea that his little girl was growing up, so when Mom started wearing makeup—lipstick and nail polish came first—he threw a fit! Mom had worked real hard at growing her fingernails out and with her own money and bought red, which was the latest fad. So one night Grandpa went in her room while she was sleeping and cut at least half of her red nails off. Then Mom started smoking and would sit out on her window and blow the smoke out so it didn't smell up her room. Mom and Duke were always on the honor roll at school, and when Mom graduated, she took the test to be a secretary for the government. During this time during World War II, they needed office workers, and the money was great. After several weeks, she received a letter. She had passed the test, and the background check was completed. So the next week, she moved in with a girlfriend and went to work in San Francisco for the FBI. She really liked the work and liked living on her own at nineteen and being self-supporting. She remembered that when the marines were in town on shore leave to watch out because they were known as "the wild bunch."

One evening, her girlfriend talked her into going on a blind date that she thought never ended up good. This is where the actual story begins. She met my dad.

When they met, I asked them what attracted them to each other. Dad first noticed her eyes; they were a brilliant blue, like the ocean. Mom commented on what a sharp-looking guy he was in his uniform, but then she got this tingle that there was something about this guy from Kansas.

After dating (remember Dad was gone a lot through 1945), it was time for Mom to bring Dad home to meet the parents. Thank heavens Duke was gone somewhere. On entering the house, they heard a commotion in the kitchen. The hot water tank had just blown and Mom's parents were on the floor, mopping as fast as they could. Mom was a little embarrassed, but Dad grabbed a rag and went to mopping; then Mom joined in, and as they were all on their knees, she introduced Dad to her parents and soon to be his in-laws. Grandpa always said that Mom found a good man, and the whole family agreed.

In May of 1946, they said their vows to each other in front of her parents and Duke. Afterward, they went out for dinner, and Dad remembered to send a telegram to his parents in Lindsborg. The Western Union telegram read this way:

> AJC4 NL PD = SAN FRANCISCO CALIF
> MAY 31 1946
>
> MR. AND MRS. FRED SUNDBERG=
> =LINDSBORG KANS=
>
> DORIS AND I MARRIED TONIGHT AT 6 PM LOVE=
>
> LOVE DORIS AND LEROY.

As you remember, Dad was stationed at Moffet Field, and shortly after they married, Flo went to visit them. Dad was leaving for a couple weeks, and they were too embarrassed to kiss in front of their visitor. She really got mad at Mom because she told her that you never let your husband leave without a kiss. You may not see him again, and that way you can say at least you had a last kiss. This was not because he was in the navy; you make that an all-time rule. She always said that this was the golden rule to marriage.

She told Mom to get out to the base, find Dad, and finish with that golden rule.

Then, several months later, they moved to Seattle, Washington, and moved close to their friends George and Helen Tubbs. In fact, George was over Dad, but they were true friends. This couple really had a lot to do with the years to come.

LT. AND MRS. LEROY SUNDBERG

Dad got his orders for the naval air base, in Seattle, Washington. He reported to his friend, Lieutenant George Tubbs, and dad's close friend since way back at the start of his Navy days. This is where dad and his crew were ordered to go and start flying to Alaska. They would transport military supplies and service personnel to bases. Dad and Mom lived in naval housing. They seemed to enjoy base housing and the different people they got to meet.

After being married for a while, mom started noticing how everyone had started their families. When they went to the beach or a barbecue at some ones house, wondering why nothing was happening for them. Finally, they found that they wouldn't be having children the natural way. They decided to put their names in to Lutheran Social Services for an adoption. Then the wait began.

GARY ANDREW SUNDBERG

The announcement read: Gary Andrew Sundberg, born April 15, 1949. Came to us on July 3, 1949.

Lieutenant and Mrs. Leroy A. Sundberg, were there firecrackers going off or what?

Back then the adoption laws had a waiting period of three to four months before the adoption began. Usually, the babies go home from the hospital to foster parents. That's the way it was with me.

When they were deciding on a name, Helen told them how to do it. Think up a bunch of names that you like, go to the back door, and stand and yell them out one at a time and see which one you like.

She said that you ended up yelling for your children three-fourths of the time, so try it out. I'm not sure if this is what Mom did, but they liked Gary Andrew Sundberg. He carried on the name Andrew, which was in all the generations before him. The only thing they didn't do was write it down and look at what the initials spelled: GAS, and this has been with him all his life, and he has it too.

From what Mom used to say about Gary, he was all boy. She said that after the day with Gary, she was so tired that she would triple his diapers and put him to bed at six-thirty p.m. But it was not a problem for Gary; he was ready for bed, and they wouldn't hear a peep out of him until around six a.m.

When he learned to crawl out of bed, they would have to be careful when they opened the door to his room because he would be asleep on the floor, looking under the crack at the bottom of the door.

Also, Gary was one of those kids who would wander off; he had the wanderlust in him. Once, they were shopping at a Penny's store, and all of a sudden, she turned around and he was gone, so she started looking for him. He had climbed into the cabinets behind the counter, slid the sliding door shut, and went to sleep. Mom really got scared when she couldn't find him, so she told a cashier and all the people employed there started yelling for him. Finally from all the commotion, he woke up and opened the door. Mom was pretty mad but so glad to find him and that he was okay. She mentioned that Gary wasn't worried; he knew where he was.

Mom finally figured out how to keep him from climbing over the fence and out of her sight. She found a halter and tied him to the clothesline. She added a little longer rope and if he were outside, she would be close. The rope was just long enough to keep away from the sides of the yard. One time, the kids from next door brought their new red wagon over and were playing with him. They thought it would be fun to give him a wagon ride. They loaded him up and away they went. Mom just happened to look up when Gary got to the end of the rope and out the wagon he flew. He thought that was fun and wanted to do it again but that was a no.

Another time, Gary was bigger, and he wanted to look through the fence at the kids next door playing in their yard. Mom felt bad and added on more rope, and Gary was satisfied watching through the fence. Then Mom ran inside to get another load of laundry out and put it on the line. When she walked back out, Gary was nowhere to be found; then Mom followed the rope, which was moving around. She got a chair and looked over the fence to find Gary hanging in his halter, but he could barely touch the ground with his tippy toes. Mom pulled him back up and over the fence, and she said that was no small feat. The rope got shortened again. He wore out several halters, but she always knew where he was. What a boy.

Dad's next base was Honolulu, and every time they were ordered to a new base, he had to take a flight test and a physical. Mom followed with Gary at her side on a ship. She said it was a nightmare because she was scared that Gary would slip away and go over the side. It was a long week, and she had to wash diapers almost every day and hang them in their cabin. They rented a house close to the beach where Dad and Mom taught him how to swim. The house was in walking distance of the base, and they loved it there and being together with Dad.

Since they were at a new base with a new squadron, Dad went to take his physical and found out there was a problem with his eye. When he was eighteen, he had been thrown from his horse and sustained a serious injury to his eye. At the time it was serious enough that the hospital sent him to Salina. He had a bad cut on the left side of his face. Well, all the flying had made the eye flare up. They tried everything at the base, but nothing worked, and Dad had to give up his service wings. He had been grounded. But it took three months to get his paperwork done, and then they offered him a teaching job at ground school, but he decided if he couldn't fly, he didn't want to be in the navy.

Mom, Dad, and Gary boarded a navy ship that was headed for the mainland and docked at San Francisco, and when they were close to docking and were headed under the Golden Gate Bridge, Gary went investigating again. The next thing they heard was the fire siren blowing, so Dad, dressed in his uniform, went up on deck to see the captain. There he found Gary, and he had pulled the siren and was being yelled at by the captain. By this time, the captain was about to yell at dad about watching his son, but he looked up and saw that Dad was higher ranked and it stopped him in his tracks. That took care of that situation. So Dad had put in ten years in the United States Naval Reserve as active duty.

When he was finally released, he had thought about getting into insurance, so he started making plans, but he decided to take his family home to visit his parents before they settled in. This is where the story takes a different turn.

THE VISIT

Dad, Mom, and Gary went back to Kansas on the train. They got off at the station in Newton, and it was very early in the morning. They knew there would be someone waiting for them, and then it would be another forty-five minutes to home.

I would guess that they were all pretty tired when they reached the farm, but I bet that Gary was excited but knew to be careful where he went. I guess that's why we always told someone where we were at or left a note in the kitchen so our parents knew where to start looking for us.

Grandpa Fred then told Dad of his plans of retiring and moving to town. Dad was shocked, and back then the oldest son took over the farm, and Fred could help out. Dad didn't say if he put pressure on him, but Ethel thought it would nice to be able to go out to the farm with the family when they were visiting. My grandparents already had bought a house, but it would be several months until they could move in. So then it was up to Mom and Dad. This was different than what they thought their future would be. The decision was made, and they took the train back and packed their possessions and moved back the next month. Dad made the comment that Mom never complained about what happened to their plans.

Back at the farm, they moved in with my grandparents, and the two families lived together for several months, and it wasn't easy. But moving day finally came, and it was one, two, three, shift. Everyone finally got settled, and life began for my parents and Gary.

The Sundberg House

Our house had seen many storms, the dust bowl days, and the Depression. It also saw three young men go off to war and then saw them come back home again. We celebrated many birthdays, Christmases, Easters, and just a lot of family reunions. It kept us safe, sound, and warm, unless the electricity went out; then we ended at Grandma and Pop's house.

It was like any other farmhouse—big, lots of rooms—it had an attic, a basement, and a washroom on the porch. The kitchen was where we ate together, but there was a dining and living room that had been separated at one time by big doors, but I can't remember who took them out. There was a den and one bathroom; Mom always wanted a bathroom upstairs, but later on, she got a big home in town.

We managed because we had to, and we didn't know any different. By this time, the house had been wired for electricity. On the front of the house was a big porch. Gary and I would use to sleep out there on hot summer nights since there was no air conditioning upstairs. Then, later on, Debby, my friend, and I would sleep out there. Mom always thought that we would have some boys meet us out on the road, but both of us will admit that we never did that.

But one night, Mom got the shock that, at the time, she deserved. Debby and I were sleeping on the porch, and all of a sudden this storm started building to the west of the house. We watched it for a while and then decided to move the bags back in on the living floor and went back to sleep. All of a sudden, that storm moved in with streaky lightning and blowing winds; then came the rain, and it poured down. We heard Mom coming down the stairs, and as she looked through the screen door, she started yelling at Dad that we weren't on the porch. She turned and looked in the living room but missed us because she didn't turn the light on, but we were sitting up, and Debby commented on Mom's baby doll pj's, and we started laughing. But Mom was on her way back upstairs to their bedroom to get Dad up. Finally, I went to the staircase and yelled up that we were sleeping on the living room floor. Debby and I always kind of wondered how they felt when they heard my voice.

Mom really fit into being a farmer's wife and mother; she made friends fairly easily and enjoyed having the neighbor ladies over for coffee. But Gary and I always will remember …

The Chicken Story: Mom vs. the Chicken

Mom always watched the way my grandma would kill a chicken for supper. She would cut the heads off and pluck their feathers and make sure the pinfeathers were pulled, and we'd have a wonderful meal for supper or the following day. It never bothered me to watch because I remember how many times that the chickens would run after me. That was scarier than seeing their heads loped off, and this was done with the fish, birds, or whatever Gary would bring home. There was an old chopped off tree that was perfect for the beheading of the bird and a small ax that was kept sharp, and the sharper, the better.

Grandma always used to say it was just her size; the quicker, the better.

Mom decided that she could do this chore, and she had even seen her own father do this. She caught a chicken and stretched the neck out, took the ax, and *whack.* First of all, she needed to keep her eyes open, and second of all, she shouldn't have screamed when she saw what happened.

She had only chopped part of the neck, and the chicken was still alive and mad. Mom let go, and the chicken flapped around and then started chasing her around the area. Gary came over to see what the commotion was. Mom was crying, and the chicken finally died. Mom told Gary that he could have the job from there on and went into the house. I wonder if she ever ate any of that bird?

WENDY MARIE SUNDBERG

I was born on August 16, 1956, and was given up for adoption, so I went to a foster home until the following October, and this is where the story begins.

In the fifties, there was an age limit for adoptive parents, and in January, Dad would have been turning thirty-five, but they went ahead and did the paperwork at the Lutheran social services in Wichita.

The phone rang, and my dad got to take the call from the social services. But Mom was working at the Fremont Church.

It was November 16 1956, and she was working on the election board. President Dwight D. Eisenhower was running for his second term as president of the United States.

When Mom got home, Dad was fixing Gary some scrambled eggs. This was one of two things that Dad could fix, after a bowl of cereal. Mom always said, "Yoohoo" as she walked in on the porch. She always hung her coat up, put away her gloves and scarf in the glove drawer across from the bathroom, and went to the bathroom. Then she went in the kitchen where her men were waiting for her. Just then, Dad asked her if she had any plans for the next day, and she said, "The usual." He asked her if she wanted to take a ride with him to Wichita; he had already made plans with Grandma for Gary to walk over to their house after school. Mom asked why he was going to Wichita, and his reply was to see their new daughter. I bet she sure was glad that she already went to the bathroom, but I do know she had to sit down at the table for a while and take the news in. They weren't prepared; all they had was a crib and a booster chair and a stroller; everything else they gave away.

My parents got to meet me the next day in Wichita. The adoption agency said that they could pick me up the next day and to get ready for me. So they went shopping for some diapers, clothes, blankets, and bottles, and everything else. Mom found out that in a couple of weeks, her friends were giving a baby shower for her and I. She always thought it was more exciting with adoption because you had nine months the other way.

November 18, 1956, I became a Sundberg, although there still was a six-month waiting period. Mom put me in a special outfit and introduced me to my aunt Dorothy, dad's sister, and Uncle Virgil. Eventually, Dorothy would be my godmother. They lived in Wichita, and my parents had to show me off.

We went to my grandparents next to show me off and meet my new brother. I couldn't go without a gift for him; I bought him a robot that he wanted, and I had such good taste. Then everyone wanted to know what they named me: Wendy Marie Sundberg. Mom said that she used to read to Gary *Peter Pan* all the time and always thought that Wendy was a different name, and Marie was the name that had been carried through the family. Ethel Marie, Dorothy Marie, etc. She also liked Trudy, but I'm really glad they decided on Wendy, and my initials don't spell a thing.

Being adopted, Gary and I never wanted to investigate, because why go mess things up? As far as we were concerned, we didn't know any different. The only thing is that the adoption center never used to get a family history. When we go to the doctor, all we have to say is that we were adopted.

Six months later, my adoption had been finalized, and Mom and Dad's names were legally put on my birth certificate. The lawyer's bill was sixty-five dollars, and when my folks moved to town, we found the cashed check in their files and in the memo place, written in dad's handwriting was, "Wendy's adoption." So the check is now in my baby book, where it belongs.

Last summer, Dean, Dad, Angie, and I went to the Eisenhower Library and Museum in Abilene, Kansas, and there is always a special memory when we come to the information about his reelection and look at the dates. I would always walk ahead and find the section and stood and waited for Dad to catch up. But when I was looking at the information they had, I always would have a lump in my throat and now a tear in my heart.

THE SUNDBERG FAMILY

Dad and Mom always made everything look easy, but it wasn't. Gary says he can remember when Mom would register everything that they bought in a book. She would sell extra eggs, milk, and cream in town for extra money. Dad was a very hard worker, but if I needed him, all I had to do is go outside and find him. Mom always said that we were lucky that his job was right outside the door. But when I was young and during the winter, Dad would get a part-time job to help ends meet. Then when I was settled in first grade, mom went to work in town until a teacher at the college talked her into working for him at his insurance agency. She went on and studied for her insurance license and became an insurance agent.

But before this, we were always on their minds; that means sometimes good and sometimes not so good.

Gary and I kind of pushed their buttons a few times and now then was okay because I have all the stories to show how they taught us about love, strength, and no matter what happened, they always loved us.

At church one Sunday morning—Mom, Dad, and Gary always sat in the north wing—Gary really had to go to the bathroom, and once church was over, our parents walked out the door, and there was Gary peeing in the bushes. Mom was mortified and all Dad had to say was, "When you got to go, you got to go."

Another time was when Mom was worried about the way Gary was slumped over when he would walk. Many times when we got home, she made him walk around with the encyclopedias on his head.

When we were young, Mom and Dad and another couple went to Kansas City for a farmers meeting, and it was cold with a cold rain coming down. The puddles filled the streets; everyone ended up with wet feet. But Mom's feet really hurt, and once they got her shoes off, her feet were so swollen and she had so much pain that she took some aspirin and kept her feet up for the rest of the weekend. Dad wanted her to see the doctor when they got home, but the pain went away. Several more times this happened, and finally she went to the doctor and was diagnosed with rheumatoid arthritis.

This was before all the new medicines that are out on the market. Then, all they had to treat it with was aspirin. Back in the late 1950s and early sixties, doctors really didn't know about it. But Mom was told that she wasn't going to die from it, but there would be days she would wish she had.

What is Rheumatoid Arthritis?

Now simply called RA, rheumatoid arthritis is a chronic disease that causes pain, stiffness, and swelling in the joints. It is an autoimmune disorder; your own body attacks the healthy tissue, causing inflammation to damaged joints. RA can be aggravated by physical activity. Sometimes your work will be hampered to the point of not being able to continue working at your job.

Did you know that one percent of the U.S. population suffers from RA? Usually people have signs of the disease appearing between the ages thirty-five to fifty, and women are affected two out of three times more than men. Mom was thirty-five and was started on massive doses of aspirin four to five times a day. This was hard on her stomach, and she got an ulcer that bled. The first time, she was at home, and the doctor wanted to admit her to the hospital because she was anemic to the point of being dangerous.

Mom was getting ready, and Dad got the car out and ready to go. The phone was ringing when he walked back in the house, and it was the doctor wondering where she was. Then Dad told him that she was putting on her makeup and that they would be there soon. Mom never went anywhere without her makeup on. She got the riot act read to her at the hospital; the doctor impressed upon her that she could bleed out in fifteen to twenty minutes, and then she would be gone.

Then Maalox came out, and being that it was new, did not come out in flavors, just that awful chalky taste, but she took it every time she would take the aspirin; the Maalox coated her stomach. She bought this by the case.

You have to remember that RA is still an incurable, inflammatory disease that progressively gets worse, and without the care from your doctor or a doctor of rheumatology, the pain will get worse, and the joints will be damaged a lot faster. Now, there are so many prescription drugs and shots that help slow and almost stop the damage, but remember that this a get-by and not a cure. Mom eventually started taking three to five milligrams of Prednisone to help bring the inflammation down and help the pain.

Mom suffered the rest of her life and had many surgeries done on her hands and feet. She had been too late for all the new medications. She told me that at night the pain got so bad that she would take a chug of whiskey to help her sleep and many times was in the hospital for pain control, or the ulcer would flare up, and many times she was given a blood transfusion.

She never complained, and it all caught up with her.

The Accident

Mom always thought that it helped to exercise, and this was the course she followed with her RA. I remember her exercising to Jack Lalanne in the mornings on the television. I remember her doing her own stretching, and she would say that's how she stayed thin, bending over and picking lint off the floor, but the more I think about her and her reactions at the time, they were due to her pain. She would read everything she could get her hands on about this horrible, painful disease, and the medical profession didn't have a lot to go on. She never complained and lived her life to the fullest.

In late May or early June, I was three years old, and she was going for a ride on Gary's bike. There was a place to sit on the back, and I remember holding on around her waist as we rode down the driveway. I had ridden with Gary many times before and learned where to hold on.

She was always so careful because of the sandy road and the country roads that had the ditches cleaned out by a road grater because a lot of sand washed off the road during the winter months. They would push the sand to the middle of the road and then even it back on the roads where it was supposed to be. This was very loose sand, and sometimes it was hard to walk on the road.

We waved to Dad as we rode out the driveway; he had pulled the combine out of the shed and started working on it for harvest in a month or two. Gary and Butch were out hunting since Mom had fixed supper early that evening. At the end of the driveway, she stopped to look both ways because vehicles drove fast on the country roads, and twilight was setting in. She didn't take any chances. So we pulled out, and everything was going fine; we were even singing a song.

All of a sudden, a dirty, ugly dog came out from the ditch and started barking at us. We were just past the mailbox, and she asked if I recognized the dog. Neither of us had, and by this time we were getting intimidated by the way the dog started growling. Every move we made, the madder the dog got, so Mom just decided to turn around and go back to the house.

As Mom made a large U-turn in the middle of the road, she told me to hang on tightly. The dog started nipping at our feet, and that's when Mom started to pedal faster, but she didn't want to kick the dog. We hit that loose sand, and we both started to fall, but the dog wouldn't leave me alone because if it nipped at my feet, I would pull them in because I was riding without shoes on. The dog finally made a move as we went down, and I naturally brought my left foot in and caught it in the spokes of the bike. I let out such a horrible scream that Dad came running, and I also scared the dog away, but the damage had already been done. I was lying in the middle of the road with Mom and bleeding all over.

Mom was yelling for help, and once Dad got there, he knew that he was going to have to ease the foot or what was left from the spoke. We used to tease him about carrying his trusty handkerchief, but it came in real handy that day because once he removed the bike, he wrapped it so tightly around my foot and told me not to look at it. Mom ran for the car, and as Dad sat with me in his arms, Mom moved the bike in the ditch and started the drive to town. Dad held me as close to him as possible. I started going into shock, and I was still bleeding to where he finally put his hand over my foot to slow down the bleeding.

Once at the hospital, they didn't leave my side, and Dad announced that he was going to surgery with me. They were using ether to knock me out. Dad was watching carefully because I had started to choke on food that was coming back up. He wasn't real sure how much of my foot was left.

Mom was in a state of shock herself, and she had gotten real scraped up; it's amazing she could drive the car. The nurses took care of her and cleaned her up, telling her that being cleaned up when I came out of surgery wouldn't scare me.

Finally, the surgery was finished, and Dad told Mom that I had lost my little toe and the toe next to it was going to be damaged the rest of my life but they left it on. There was a cut that went from the side, inward and deep. One hundred stitches went into closing the foot; lots were in the inside, and I had a bandage that went up pretty far on my leg. Mom stayed the night with me, and I spent it throwing up from the ether, which was a horrible side effect.

Dad remembered Gary, and it was almost dark. Gary and Butch had gotten back to an empty house and no note. Gary knew something was wrong and waited for a phone call, which finally came. Dad told him what happened and thought that he better get his bike out of the ditch. Being really upset, he went out to get the bike and was shocked by all the blood, and there was tissue from my foot still in the spokes. He got very angry, so he put Butch on the porch and loaded his gun and started looking for the dog. Butch wanted to go but would be safer on the porch. He started tracking the dog, and the path led him through the hedge roll and out into the pasture that he knew like the back of his hand. He found the dog and realized that the dog was sick as he watched from many feet away. He raised the gun and put the dog out of its misery. He brought the carcass to the barn in case the dog needed to be tested for rabies. Dad came home soon after Gary got back in the house and cleaned his gun. He told Dad that he took care of the dog and that he had brought the dog to the barn, but there had been no bites on Mom or me, so he and Dad buried the dog together. The next afternoon, Gary and Dad came to visit, and Gary brought me what looked like Pluto from the Walt Disney show that we watched on Sunday evenings, and I loved it. In fact, his name was Pluto. I never knew that Gary had taken care of the dog until many years later. When I got to go home, I was carried around a lot, and Mom took a picture of me outside on a blanket in the yard or in the lawn chair with my foot up high. Dad carried me upstairs to bed as he always did, but he put his arm around me just a little tighter than usual. Mom made sure that I had the right foods to build up my blood, but I never knew about the nightmares she had, and she always felt that she was at fault, but I never thought she was; she did the best thing she could do in that situation. Finally, being old enough, she told me about the nightmares, and once in a while, she still had them, just like it happened that day. But I remember that she would cuddle with me and stroke my hair, and with every stroke I always knew she loved me. I remember the last time she stroked my hair, I had fallen asleep by the side of her hospital bed with my head in my arms leaning against the mattress; I was woken with her running her finger through my hair a few days before we had to say good-bye.

As for Pluto, Angie, my daughter, fell in love with him and couldn't wait to get to her grandparents house, and he is now living at her home where she and her husband live. So Pluto lives on.

STORIES ABOUT THE FARM

Farming is not an easy way to make a living, but Dad made it look easy. Gary and I started out with the same routine of chores. Then the older we got, the more responsibility was given to us. We used to try to take shortcuts, but in the end, Dad would always find out, and we could never figure out what his secret was.

The farm made us a good living, there were hard times, but when the seventies came along, Dad really did well.

The following stories are a few that I picked out; our parents showed us a lot about farming and the strength you have in the game of life. We didn't know that's what they were preparing us for; we just thought it was work.

The farm was made up with different projects depending on the seasons of the year. There were a lot of four-legged animals on our farm; the cattle were the income, and they were taken care of with the utmost care and Dad saw to that. We all worked together, and sometimes strange things happened. When the cattle were driven up to summer pasture, we would turn to harvesting wheat, alfalfa, milo, and corn. We baled a lot of hay and put up silage in the silo while the cattle were back for the winter months.

In between those times we would put in a large garden for us that started the day after Easter. Dad would use the equipment and work the ground and would cultivate the area where Grandpa had always put down his potatoes. This was always our family project during the summer.

The Family Garden

As I said before, the family garden was very important to us. We had fresh vegetables for very little money. The Sundbergs always had a large garden in the orchard where we also had several fruit trees—apple, pear, and cherry—and I still hate pitting cherries.

After Easter, we started planning, and Grandpa would already be out preparing the ground for the potatoes. He loved planting potatoes, and once he had them in the ground, he would cultivate and work the ground until the plants came up. He would put hay around the plants to keep the moisture in the ground, and then he'd wait.

Dad would always hook the plow to the tractor and run it through the garden several times and dump a load of cow manure in the ground and plow it under.

When Gary was older, he did the planning, roping of the garden, and deciding where everything would go. He would study the seed catalog like it was the Bible. Then he'd start making the order, and on every order he got to pick something different, and sometimes he grew some strange things. With the help of Grandpa, we planted pumpkin seeds, and the important thing is that you don't plant them the usual way. There is a special way, and we really had a pumpkin patch. Gary and I sold them to the grocery store for Halloween and made enough money for Christmas gifts. That was a special Christmas Eve because everyone knew how important it was and where the pumpkin money went.

Radishes were always the first to go in because they grew so fast that you could plant several plantings until midsummer. When you bit into one, it was hot. We planted tomatoes, green beans, peas, carrots, chard, green peppers, onions, cucumbers, lettuce, okra, and beets. Planting was always fun, but weeding was not my favorite. When the plants took over, there was less weeding.

We really had a lot of produce. Grandma enjoyed coming out and helping Mom with the freezing and the canning, and she was also back in her kitchen where she once had fixed many a meals for her young family. We shared everything with my grandparents, even when Dad butchered, they got to fill their freezer up too. This is family; we provide for everyone. It was neat to plan the noon meal and go out and pick whatever you needed early in the morning. New potatoes and snap green beans were always my favorite.

All the canning jars and onions and sometimes

garlic would be in the pantry room down in the basement. In October, Mom would always buy a hundred pounds of potatoes to fill us up during the winter because Mom always knew how to make comfort food. Of course, she made it look so easy.

Gary and I would carry everything down to the basement. The pantry was a small room, and we had two cabinets and a table; the potatoes were kept on the floor so they didn't rot, and what was left over after Easter, Grandpa and Gary would cut up and plant, eyes down. Garlic and onions would hang from the pipes, so we had almost everything we needed.

Baking Day

Fridays were always Mom's baking day; she would bake rye bread, white, and would do the baking for Sunday's meal. There were always cupcakes for lunches and cookies. She made the best chocolate chip cookies, and I learned from the best. These were hand mixed and homemade. She would seal everything when it was cooled down and put into the freezer on the back porch, so if we needed anything we could just grab it. She used to make cinnamon rolls in the winter, and they were the best. Everyone always laughed because when she brought a cake somewhere, there was always a slice out of it. Guess who? Dad.

When I think back to those days, my best memory was when Gary was in high school and was center on the football team. Before a game, he would come home for a snack; he would cut the heels off the end of the loaves, and Mom would tell him not to. She said it would dry the loaf out, but how did she know? We still ate it.

Anyway, she would always tell Gary not to get hurt because she would have to come down to the field and see how he was. He told her that she better not, but he knew she would never do that.

We went to all his games, home and away. We were at Lyons, Kansas, and it was blowing and snowing. We would sit with blankets on, and of course Mom always brought hot chocolate, coffee, and cookies along. We would bring paper sacks to put our feet in for insulation. This was the night I saw my parents scared when all the players got up from the pile and there was a player down on the field, Gary. They watched as the coaches ran out on the field, and they had to help him off the field, and the pain he was in wasn't good. When Gary got his senses back, he saw Dad there. He started to say something, but Dad stopped him in midsentence and said that Gary never told him that he couldn't come down on the field. Gary's shoulder was out of place; the coaches thought they got it back in, and Gary wanted to ride home on the team bus, so we followed them back to Lindsborg, and then we end up in the emergency room. The doctor had to redo the shoulder.

The 3 Ds: Dad, Dean, and Duchess

Gary had two Irish setters; the male was Red, and the female was Duchess, and somehow we inherited her.

She was very active, and you would have thought that she would have picked Mom over Dad since Mom was the one that brushed her and cut the burrs out of her red coat.

She loved to go bye-bye in the truck with Dad, so if he went to look at a field, she was sitting in her seat in the truck. One time, Dad was looking at a field to see if it was ready to cut, and she was running around. She went to the neighbors' house and was laying on their front porch in the shade. The problem was that the people had just painted the porch, so the next day, Dad went and repainted the porch, and Duchess ran around with a painted belly.

There were times when she thought that Dad was ignoring her, especially when he was working on the farm equipment. Dad would always lay out the tools he needed so he could just reach without looking. Duchess would lie under the equipment, and after awhile she would take off with a screwdriver or pliers or whatever, and there was Dad, trying to find the tool. He knew, so he would crawl back out and chase her, which she loved, but he was mad. Somewhere on that farm, there are tools that are buried.

Dad won a farming award and was going to be honored at a banquet; they wanted pictures, and I was supposed to rush home from school. Well, I didn't make it, but Duchess was there to take my place. It was a great picture.

Dean found out the hard way when he was playing with her. She was chasing him around the barn yard. What he didn't know was she always gets her man. Those long legs and large feet tripped him up, and he went down and sprained his ankle. He didn't run from her again.

Harvesting

When the cattle were in the summer pasture and we knew they were all right, it was time to get the combine and trucks ready for harvesting. The end of June was the start of a very busy time of the year. First was harvesting the wheat. We didn't mess around, because you walked lightly around Dad until the wheat crop was in. You worried when the crop was almost ready and the heads were getting heavy and started leaning over; you knew it would take one good thunderstorm with pea-sized hail to destroy your entire wheat crop. Another worry toward the end is rain. Around May, those simple spring rains are much needed. We never seem to worry about the milo crop or the corn crop because the milo is very hardy, and the corn was irrigated, and you have many months before those fields are ready, usually October. We were always busy with having enough hay and feed on hand when we brought the cattle home for the winter. My dad said just the other day, "You have one hundred head of cattle; you have a hundred problems."

We never cut in the morning because the wheat was damp from the evening, and we didn't like when we were docked for moisture from the Farmer Union Elevator. So we would get up early, cut, bale and stack alfalfa. Then, as the morning progressed, we would check out the trucks engines because you didn't want them overheating in the field. Fires were something else to worry about. Gary taught me how to do maintenance. Dad had our hired hand out plowing a field that had just been cut. Grandpa always loved to help until his eyes got bad. So it was up to Mom and me to take over the job of driving to town with a load of wheat. We never had an accident because we were careful and always remembered to stop and look twice both ways when we were coming out of the field to the road. This was our income we were hauling. But the last load of the season, Dad always took to town.

The mornings were early, and we got started in the fields around noon. We worked until sunset; Dad was never one to work in the fields at night. There was only one time that I remember; there was a thunderstorm, and they were predicting severe winds and hail. We worked very late on getting a field done by the house so that the equipment could be taken home and put away. The storm came, and we ended up in the basement late that night.

When everyone was home and bathed and Dad had figured the tickets that we got with each load, Dad always loved to have root beer floats for supper, and then he was off to bed. In the morning it was "rise and shine," and we were off for another day. I never went to town during harvest because I knew Dad was relying on my help. I often would take a book with me and read in the truck until he was ready for another load.

Mom had her jobs; during the year, she would collect gallon jugs and wrap them with burlap. Each one of us had our own jugs for water, and the burlap kept the water cool. She would always fix a big turkey, and we had sack lunches out in the field. Being in the heat, and it was hot, we didn't want very much to eat. Eating wasn't on our minds at the time.

In 1972, the harvest was great, and Dad decided it was time for some new equipment. For him, it was a new combine that had a cabin with air. The radio was AM/FM, and there was room if someone wanted to ride along. It was time that Dad had new equipment, and when he would come in at night, he wasn't dirty anymore. He bought a new big truck that he could haul wheat and cattle in. I thought this was heaven after mom and I learned how to drive it in high and low gears, double clutching. We drove it around the mile line to make sure we knew what we were doing. This truck probably could haul at least two to three loads more than what the pickup trucks hauled. You could push a button and the back would rise up and unload itself. The best part was the air conditioner, cassette player, and the AM/FM radio. I never used the air condition when I had a load; I thought that it might be too much on the engine. We were working in style.

Mom and I were so scared that we would put the first dent in the truck, knowing that Dad didn't have time to enlarge the door on the barn. So you would have to stop and pull in the big mirror on the side and then drive in. We made sure of this every night.

It was the last load of the season, and Dad was excited about getting to finally drive the truck. We had all the equipment home, and Mom always fixed something special and we would have iced tea and munchies on the patio when Dad arrived home. He always honked the horn all the way down the driveway for having a successful and safe harvest. He drove on down to the shed when, all of a sudden, we heard this horrible crash.

We ran to see what happened, and as Dad came walking out of the shed, and he was okay, we saw those two large mirrors on the ground, both lying in a pile. No one dared to laugh, and he wasn't too happy with himself.

The next morning, while he took the truck in to order new mirrors, Grandpa, Gary, and GW were worked on enlarging the shed doors.

Dad has been out of farming for years, but another farmer is renting the ground that was handed down through the generations. Dad really appreciates this man and his family because pretty soon his family will be working in the fields, just like we did, and I have noticed how he farms so much like my father did. They are so considerate about getting my dad so he can ride the combine with his renter while he is working on our fields.

THE FARM KIDS

At school we were known as "the farm kids." We had to bring our sack lunches while the city kids got to go home for lunch. This lasted until we were freshmen in high school; then we got to eat in the cafeteria.

But at home, there were chores to be done. Dad always did the morning chores because when busing started up, we needed to be out at the end of the driveway early.

Gary and I both had special animals that we cared for and were our responsibility. Butch the dog was Gary's best friend, and when Gary got his gun out or his fishing rod out, she was so excited that she just couldn't wait.

The Hunting Buddies

One day, a light brown dog that was kind and built like a beagle, came up to us while Gary and I were doing something by the house. It was another dog that someone didn't want and dumped out in the country to fend for herself. She was so hungry and thirsty that Mom put some leftovers and water out for her. When Dad came home, we didn't honestly know how he would feel, and he hated when a stray dog would be dropped off because he would usually have to shoot it before it got rabies or it became mean. But after looking her over and petting her, we knew we had a dog. We fixed up a box that we made cozy for her, and at night, Gary figured out how to keep the door open in case she needed to go out.

Being so excited about having another dog, I was the first one out the next day. As I opened the door, she growled at me. So I went to get Gary, and she did the same thing to him. Suddenly, she saw it was Gary, and he knew exactly what the problem was; she had a couple puppies in the night. Once she knew we wouldn't hurt her or her puppies, she was glad to see us. We started really pushing the food and water. We wanted to touch the puppies so bad but thought we shouldn't until their eyes opened and they were running after Butch. Dad wasn't real thrilled about the whole ordeal but knew if we voted, it would be three to one. When the puppies were weaned, we found homes for them, except one. I had fallen for a puppy, and Dad let me keep him; his name was Dino, after the Flintstones. Dino was kind of a strange dog and took to Dad more than me. He loved to follow Dad out to the field and stay there until he was done, but one day, Dad came home without Dino. He was disking the field, and Dino was chasing a rabbit and under the disk they both went. Dad said that he didn't suffer, and he buried both the animals by the hedgerow and made sure that no animal would dig them up by placing rocks over the grave. He was so upset; he never liked to see an animal die. So he and I both mourned the rest of the day.

Butch, on the other hand, was taken to the vet and was fixed, so this didn't happen again. Butch became one of the family; she was a good dog but very loyal to Gary. Their friendship was very touching.

If we had been away from the house, she would show us that she had been on duty when we drove in and deserved a treat. She was always invited into the kitchen for a cookie. She knew to sit pretty and really loved Mom's chocolate chip cookies. But if we had bought cookies, she wasn't impressed but took them anyway.

She hated thunderstorms, and so she was under the washer and felt safe. The washing machine dripped oil and it would drip on her back. This got to be a permanent spot, because she didn't like fireworks either.

One day, after the chores were done, Gary decided to go in the hay meadow and do some hunting before supper that evening. He told Mom where he would be, and out the driveway, Gary and Butch, with that wagging tail, left on an adventure.

When supper was on the table, Dad yelled for Gary, but he never came, so we went ahead and ate, but I could see the concern in their eyes, and Gary wouldn't have missed a meal unless something went wrong. While Mom and I were cleaning off the dishes and washing them, I saw Dad go outside and start looking around until we saw him take off running down the drive way. He saw Gary with Butch around his neck and full of blood. Gary was in tears and told Dad that he had accidentally shot her.

He was aiming at some birds, and as he went to aim, he lost track of Butch, and usually she would stay behind until he took a shot. But she was trying to help him by flushing them out. The next thing we knew, Dad came in told Mom to call the vet cause Butch was alive but had been shot. He grabbed his keys and away they went. We came to find out that the bullet broke her front right leg and then lodged in her chin; she still had to have surgery, and she had lost a lot of blood, so she had to spend the night. The first thing the next morning, Dad and Gary went to pick up Butch, and she was her old self, except with a cast. Mom fixed her up a corner in the kitchen, and boy did she get the attention.

A couple weeks later, we saw Gary walking down the driveway and Butch following on three legs and one cast sticking out in front.

Butch died of old age on the farm, and Dad buried her out in the pasture where she loved to run, and he saw to it that her grave was covered with lots of rocks.

Gary had lost the best buddy he ever had.

My Horse Named Daisy

Daisy was living at the farm before I was, but we became buddies when I was older. Dad would always walk her around with me on her back.

I rode her a lot. All I would have to do was call to her and bang on a bucket with oats in it and that enticed her to come to me. While she would eat her oats, I would bridle her and bring her over to a wood fence and jump on her back, and off we went. This didn't always go real smooth because I would sometimes jump a little farther than I needed and jumped over her and fell to the ground. She would always turn her head and look at me sitting on the ground, and I bet you know what she was thinking, but I felt real stupid.

She was a good kid horse, and many kids rode her. She was the highlight of many birthday parties. Mom always worried that I didn't spend enough time with my girlfriends in grade school and wanted me to have them overnight. But most of my friends wanted to ride horses and that's all. I don't think that I ever told her about this.

Daisy did her share of the work; we always had cattle drives twice a year, in the spring around Easter and in October before winter set in.

The neighbors and us always took a Saturday where we would saddle the horses and go on a cattle drive. There were usually around eight on horseback, and Grandpa would throw bales in the back of the truck and park it where the cows would see him and follow him on the road to the driveway into the pasture. Usually, rounding them up into a herd was the hardest part, and sometimes they weren't very happy with us.

The summer pasture was probably five miles up in the hills, and this took longer than you might think.

This pastureland had everything that the cattle needed, lots of grassland and a pond for drinking and cooling off. When they were brought home for the winter, they would have a tank that we would pump fresh water to and break the ice when needed.

Daisy was a good cow horse because she would know how to watch their heads on which way they were going, but in the end, she would change their minds and get back on track.

The only thing that she didn't like was the blanket and the saddle, but Dad insisted on this because it saved her back, and the riders were safer too. But when it was over, she knew that I would brush her down while she ate her oats.

One late afternoon, Dad and I rode up to bring home a sick cow and her calf. Dad's brother was visiting and drove the truck to the entrance of the pasture. Now, this cow would spook real easy, and we decided that Dad would take it slow and kind of move both of the animals up the side of the hill by the fence. Then, once on the hill, I would take over and herd them slowly down to where Charles was with the truck. Sounds easy, doesn't it?

Well, that was a dream. Things were going well until the cow was spooked almost to the top, and she went another way around the hill, so Daisy and I took off on the top of this rocky hill when Daisy tripped, and we both went down. But Daisy got back up, and as she stood, her front hooves caught my hand, and I was really hurt and I didn't want to move. Daisy looked down at me; she knew, and she stayed there until Dad saw her. I remember his horse climbing the hill with a gallop.

Dad looked me over and knew right away that there was something wrong with my hand, so he put me back on Daisy and led his horse and Daisy down the hill to the truck and told Charles to get me to Mom. Mom called the doctor and took me down to his office. He X-rayed my hand and cleaned up all the places where the rocks cut me. He said I was very lucky that I had jeans on, but I probably wouldn't be wearing them again, and my hand wasn't broken, just smashed. There was no cast, but a sling, ice, and heat. He also told me no horseback riding until he X-rayed my hand in two weeks. As for the pants, that was one of Dad's rules: no riding the horse without jeans on. Then Dad came through the door, and he had to walk both horses home because he couldn't lead and hold on to his own horse.

When I got home, I went to see if Daisy was all right. She had a few nicks on her, and Dad made sure her hooves were okay. Then he put cream on her cuts and gave her a double amount of grain. I brought her a carrot and sugar that came in cubes; those were her two favorites.

The next day, Dad, Charles, and Grandpa brought the cow and calf home and down to the vet to be taken care of.

Daisy was a good friend until Dad found her in the pasture, and she had died of old age. He had her taken off before I got home from school, and I know she died knowing all the secrets we shared, and she never told them to anybody. I still have a memory of her and the breast belt that went with her saddle and briddle. I think of her now and then, but she has a special place in my heart.

Fun on the Farm

Gary and I had a lot of fun on the farm, even though he liked to tease me and then I would yell. Our parents always advised me on two different facts. One, he wouldn't tease me if he didn't like me, and besides I yelled good. Two, you always know who ends up getting hurt.

I asked Gary one time about how he felt about me coming into his life after he had been the center of attention for seven years. He was excited about having a sister, and it never seemed to bother him. I once found a saying in a book: "It was nice growing up with someone like you, someone to lean on, someone to count on, someone to tell on." This was the way it was at the Sundberg farm. Our parents always had to stay two steps ahead of us at all times.

Gary always found a way to pick on me, and most of the time, I deserved it. When we were in the backseat of the car, there was a seam that went down the middle of the seat, and he dared me to cross it, and, of course, I did, and then he would whoop me. The problem was that I was too stubborn to quit, and pretty soon my hand was awful red.

Yes, I bothered him a lot and probably was a pain, but he used to run upstairs to bed before me. Upstairs, there was a long, dark hallway that led to another bedroom that we used as the storeroom. He waited for me to come up the stairs, and then he ran down the hallway and scared me; I screamed. Then one of our parents would end up upstairs and tried to get me to bed. But Gary got told to go to his room. But he was always there, especially on cold winter mornings when the ice was thick on the inside of our windows. I would run and climb in his bed; he was always so warm, like a big heating blanket, and he always let me stay there with him.

He and I had lots of adventures together, and to this day, we still have adventures, but our parents aren't there to make peace. We had a great time on the farm, well, at least lots of memories that we laugh at now.

The Bucket System

Gary and I were just like any kids. We tried to get away with as much as possible, and if there were any shortcuts, we would figure out a way.

The evening was coming on, and one of our chores was to feed the cattle that were up in the corral near the barn and put grain in the feeders. Well, we had messed around too long, and Mom had just called us in for supper. So my job was to get in the room where the grain was and scoop grain in the buckets for Gary. Then he would carry them out to the cows. These were five-gallon metal buckets with handles.

When we finally finished, we decided not to put the buckets back in the grain room but left them outside by the barn door. We were hungry and cold, and in the house we went.

We thought that since it was Friday evening, we would just get up a little early and get the buckets and start our morning chores before Dad was out. We promised that we would not tattle on each other. This was our first mistake.

The evening went on, and we were ready to hit the sack and proud of ourselves that we had gotten away with something. We were in our own rooms when Mom yelled for us, and we figured that we had forgotten to brush our teeth. Mom always felt our toothbrushes, and if they were dry, well, you know how that ended.

When we got downstairs in our pj's, robes, and slippers—mine were pink fuzzy slippers—Dad asked if there was something that we had forgotten. As we looked at each other, we knew we were had. So we got our coats, hats, and mittens over our pj's, and Dad handed us a flashlight as we walked out the door. Off we went in the night, which was real scary, and there were lots of noises I had never heard. Once we got to the barn, Gary opened the sliding, wood door, and we both put the buckets in where they belonged in the first place and shut the door behind us and ran back to the house. Of course, Gary had the flashlight, and he could outrun me and I screamed all the way to the house.

The next morning at breakfast, Dad explained why the metal buckets need to be in the barn at night. When its cold out, they will rust and that is not good to feed the cattle with rusted buckets. Well, we understood what he was saying, and we each had an extra job that day. But what we couldn't understand was how did he know?

Getting Back

Gary got away with so many things, and I always seemed to get the worst of the deal, but this next story I figured out a way to get back at him.

We both learned to drive at an early age, and besides, what could go wrong out in the pasture in first gear? This is where Dad loaded up the truck with hay bales and fed the cattle. I drove, and Gary would be in the back, pulling the string that was around the bales, and he'd pull the bale apart and throw it out the back for the cattle, and they always knew what time it was. When the truck pulled through the gate, it was suppertime.

I had learned how to pop the clutch, and the truck would jerk, so I waited till Gary was at the end of the truck to pop the clutch, and out the back of the truck he went on his bottom. I stopped the truck and asked what happened very innocently. He didn't really comment. I asked him if he was okay, and he was. So we went back to feeding, and I waited, and at the right time, I popped the clutch again and out the back he went again. Now, I thought this was funny and I wonder if that is why he has a bad back.

One night, Gary was doing something else for Dad, and he said that he would feed the cattle, and, as usual, I drove. Once out in the pasture, I thought that I would show my trick to Dad. I then popped the clutch and out the back Dad went on his bottom. It was funny up to the point that I found out that he landed in a warm, fresh, pile of cow poop. Boy, was I in trouble, and I never did that again.

Gary thought it was so funny; he had been hoping that I would do my trick with Dad in the back. I will always wonder why I did that to Dad.

Later on, I found out that I really didn't need to be in the truck because when the truck was in first gear, it would just go on its own without a driver. Dad just thought that this was something I could do.

Gary's New BB Gun

One year, Dad had decided to put all new windows in the barn. He was getting ready because the barn usually was a very busy place. The stalls would be cleaned, and new hay was laid for a hay bed. The heat lights were checked, and any other necessities were ready to go.

Gary had gotten a new BB gun for Christmas, and of course he already knew how to use it. Dad and my grandpa Oscar always made sure that Gary knew how to carry a loaded gun and other rules. So we went out around the barnyard looking for something to shoot at.

I didn't ever use his BB gun because on his first gun, he was teaching me to aim and fire, except I had my finger in the wrong place and ended up losing my fingernail. The doctor had to drill through the nail to take the pressure off and help the pain. But I always thought it was nice to be asked to go. We were having a great time and decided to shoot at the windows in the barn. We didn't know that Dad had replaced them and that they were new. What fun we had; at least every window had at least one hole in it. Good shooting, until Dad heard the glass breaking and then noticed that the windows had been shot out of the frames. All the windows that had holes had to be replaced because they had been weakened and eventually would break out due to the cold and wind. I told him that we didn't do it, but we thought they were still broken and that was my first mistake. My second mistake was that I said that we sure had fun.

No BB gun, and when our parents took something away from us, they never gave us a date when we would see it again. We had to work and show some responsibly before we earned the gun back. We also lost our allowance and knew not to ask when we would start getting it back, and extra chores had been added to the list, and if Dad didn't have something for us to do, he would send us to Mom in the house, and she always had something for us to do.

Dad and Grandpa replaced the windows again, but I have never seen Dad that mad at us.

It was another learning experience to put away in our memories.

The House Up the Road

My dad would always extend farming by renting farmland from farmers who had decided to retire or a person who received land through an estate. One piece of land happened to be up on the next mile line. He planted wheat and had pastureland on the other side, but there was an old house on this property that was just waiting for the family to come back. I have noticed that when a house doesn't have a family living in it and there is no love, it simply dies.

When Dad went up to do some work, Gary and I always wanted to go because there was a secret that we found in the house. There had been a golf course on part of the pasture, and you could still see where the greens were, but it got harder to see with time. The weeds and wildflowers had taken over their domain. But cattle enjoyed every bit of it.

The house was bigger than our house and was built by that same builder that built our house. But he really put a lot more work in this house; because of all the woodworking and beautiful carved patterns on the doors, he must have gotten more money, and I think our house was older. Dad always said that the house was built better for its time.

We always entered through the back porch, which was called the mudroom. Next, you entered the kitchen, and it was kind of like ours because they must have eaten all their meals there unless they had company, in which case they used their dining room. But the strange thing was that the table was set with the dishes and a tablecloth deteriorating under the dishes where once covered with food but had been eaten through the years. Someone had done the chores because the wood box by the stove had been filled, waiting for the next meal to be fixed. The pie cabinet didn't have a drop of food that was meant to be cooling; on the sides of the cabinet was a design of small holes from top to bottom to cool the goodies off from the day's baking. The dishes were all in their place but, through the time, were dusty. I would suppose that there had been some thankful critters that enjoyed all the food that had been left out.

The next room was the best because it was decorated and beautiful. The dining room was a room that when the occupants had company, this is where they would have been served. The large table had six chairs that were all ready for company, and the coal light was filled and hung perfectly over the table; it reminded me of a prism with the west sun making its presence known to the room. The dining room had a beautiful buffet with the good dishes, which were dull from not being used.

Their company would have entered though the front door and were welcomed by the beautiful walnut staircase. I remember playing with the large sliding doors that closed off the front room to the dining room and that still slide with ease. The front room had beautiful windows that used to keep the winds from the south at bay. This would have been an excellent place for plants, and the large doors were made for privacy or entertaining guests.

Their coats were still hung with care on the front hallstand with a framed mirror waiting to show the family how they looked as they left their home. Now, the coats that had kept the family warm were now nice warm homes for the spiders that had a large web over the mirror.

The grand walnut staircase still had a slight shine and was built with a kid in mind. But, being a girl, I could imagine my dad and I coming down the stairs as the bride and her father as her escort. The staircase now would creak and moan as you made the turn on the landing and up another four stairs. This led to the four bedrooms and our secret. There were two bedrooms made up alike, ready to have someone settle down for the night. The beds were made, and the oil lights were full and ready to be read by. Each had lace doilies that were handmade, like my grandma taught me to make. They all matched the scarves that were on the dressers in the room. I remember the lights by both beds were beautiful glass. The dresser drawers were pulled out like someone was in a big hurry and forgot to push them in again.

Down the hallway was another room, although very small. This looked like they were in the process of fixing it up like a library, but the shelves had not been built. The books were sitting on the floor and had been stacked as if organized at one time. The old Sears catalog books were fun to look at, and we used to call them our "wish books." There also was a large walk-in closet, which was different at the time. The wire hangers were still in all the closets, waiting to have clothes hung on them, as if they had just been washed and ironed.

The fourth bedroom must have belonged to a child because this is where the secrets were. The bed was made, but it looked like they had been reading comic books and then pushed them off the bed. Gary and I enjoyed reading them since we only got one when we had been sick so Mom could keep us in bed or for a birthday gift. If Gary and I tried to read all the comics, we would have been reading a couple hours everyday for months. This was in the middle sixties, if not earlier, but Gary enjoyed reading them to me. To us, this room had been our gold mine.

Then Dad would yell for us, and it was time to go home; then we would give the staircase a much-needed dusting as we slid down the banister. It was a great ride, and our bottoms showed it.

As we walked out through the mudroom, I always turned around and looked at the braided rugs on the floor and wondered how much smaller they would be the next time because the rats or some critter pulling them apart, probably making their nest somewhere. My grandma used to make those kinds of rugs out of leftover rags, jeans, or material that was left over when Mom was sewing.

Through the years, the weather started beating down the house and was winning. Dad started to cover the broken windows with sheets of metal; at least that helped a little bit.

We never knew what happened in that house or who had once lived there, but I'm sure there is a story about it. We always wanted to take some of the comic books home to read, but Dad always said no. They didn't belong to us, and we had to put them back in the room where we had found them.

To my knowledge, nobody ever returned to live in the house, and one morning when Dad went to do the chores, he smelled something suspicious in the wind. He looked over, and the house was gone and what was left was still smoldering. The house had finally died, but it must have been a glorious ending. What used to be a lovely old house turned to nothing but ashes. It was never known how the fire was started, and to this day, I will drive by where the driveway once was and now has disappeared and is covered by a wheat field, and the steel windmill that once stood tall is almost gone. So you can still see that there had been a homestead there at one time.

But Gary and I always enjoyed our big playhouse and the entertainment that our secret of the house up the road held. The house at least knew that we once loved it and that will always stay between Gary and me.

MOTHER NATURE AT HER BEST

Living on a farm was busy all year round, and the cattle made it very interesting, especially during the calving season. The cattle naturally knew what to do, thanks to Mother Nature. But sometimes the weather would get in the way, and we would have to step in and help. We never lost too many calves, but there were times we had close calls.

When we brought the cattle home from summer pasture, we may have already had some new calves. But it seemed like between January through March was really busy. Dad and Grandpa, with the help of Gary and I, would clean up the stalls in the barn and lay hay, thick and fresh on the floor. We made sure the heating lamps were ready and would try to put most the cows who were due closer to the house, but sometimes we would miss one, and when the weather was nasty cold, the calves were born wet, and the cow couldn't clean them off in time before they would freeze to death. So we would intervene and take the calf and mother to shelter. Usually the mother would follow when you picked up her calf, and she gave us no trouble, like she knew we were trying to help.

Mom's kitchen would become a nursery and the basement did too. We would turn on the stove and open the door and start rubbing them down to dry them off and stimulate the calves. Gary and Dad would work on calves down the basement under a heat light and would make a bed near the furnace. We would put old towels on the floor and let them suck on our fingers. Mom had one rule: As soon as they started to stand and walk around, it was time for them to go back to their mom. We would take them back to the barn where the mother was, and they usually were ready to nurse.

By the next day, they were usually ready to go back to the herd, and we would get ready for the next round. Working together, we probably saved more calves and it seems we always worked harder on little bulls.

Bottle Feeding

There were times when the calves would need to be bottle-fed. Dad or Mom would mix up the formula for us, and the bottles were nothing like a baby bottle. They were big enough to hold with two hands, and I'm not sure how much it held, but the thing I remember the most was how bad it smelled. They had a long nipple, kind of like a tit of a cow, and the calves would nudge it and bump it with their heads like they did with their moms. Sometimes they would pull the nipple off the bottle and the formula would spray out, and once it got on you, you would smell for the rest of the day.

There were some cows that didn't want to nurse or maybe their mothers died in birth. Dad would work with them and another cow to make the calf nurse and that was no easy task. We kept the cow and the calf together, and Dad would put the cow in the loading shoot and put a fence between him and her. Then he was handed the calf and showed the calf where to nurse, and the calf was ready to eat—that wasn't the problem; it was always getting the cow to hold still. We would have some successes and failures, but knowing Dad, he always had something up his sleeve.

Gary's Piglets

Gary was in an after-school club called FFA (Future Farmers of America), and he had to have a project his junior and senior year. One year was pigs, and he bought a pig that already was pregnant because he wanted to start out with piglets, and he got his money's worth.

The pig had around ten babies, and it took all of us to help; she shot them out so fast that Gary would help deliver them and cut the cords and hand them to us. We would clean them off and put them in bushel baskets, three to a basket. She started to nurse them when she was done having them.

Once they were running around, we moved mom and babies back to the place that Gary made for them.

They grew really fast, and they were fun to play with when the mother wasn't up.

Gary told me how I played with three piglets, and I taught them how to sit, stand on their back legs, follow me in a line, and some other little tricks. Of course, when they did their tricks, they were rewarded with food, and believe me, I don't ever think they got full. Gary brought Dad over to the pigpen when I was playing with them and showed Dad how I had trained them. He just shook his head, but they were really easy to train. I don't think that's what Gary had in mind for his project.

Watching that pig give birth was pretty exciting; it almost looked like a ballet. I was so thrilled Gary let me help and care for his pigs. The only bad part of the day was that we were up early with the birthing, and then we had to go to school. Gary used my camera, the Swinger from Kodak, and it was one of the new cameras that you pulled the film out and counted to ten and the picture would be developed. He wanted to show his FFA teacher.

Gary took his hogs to market and sold them and made good money on them that went into his savings. Everything that we earned off our animals went in to a savings account.

We had a lot of animals; Donald and Daisy were our two ducks until Mom made us get rid of them because they always pooped on the sidewalk to the house. Then Gary had rabbits and sold them around Easter. Never a dull moment …

Checking on the Cattle

During the summer after a thunderstorm, Dad always wanted to check on the cattle in the summer pastures. This was always a good time because when it rained everything came to a halt in the field. So we would saddle up the horses in the early morning so we could be back by eleven, before the heat came on.

We would go and count the cattle from afar so they wouldn't move around; then we would walk the horses through the herd to make sure they weren't hurt or sick. If our count didn't come out right, we would ride the whole pasture for fear that one of the herd got struck by lightning. Then we would see if there were any new calves.

The horses always knew when we were headed for home because they usually wanted to run back, and we held them back so we didn't fall in a hole. One horse that we had was really strange. Every time he would go through water, he always had to roll or just sit down, and he didn't care who was on his back. Buck was a really handsome stud, but we never knew what he was up to. One day, he hadn't given my dad any trouble, and we crossed a creek that had overflowed its bank. Daisy and I crossed with no problem until I turned around and Buck sat down in the middle, and I saw Dad sliding off his back into the water. Once he was back on land with Buck, he ended up soaked to the skin, and Buck acted like nothing happened. Dad said a few choice words on the matter, and I knew not to laugh; the timing wasn't good. Those were great times, and Dad said that this is how he had time for me since I wasn't around following him everywhere. I know I missed those times.

DAD'S HIRED HELP

Dad would usually have to hire juniors or seniors to help with the baling and other little jobs. Then he would also have a young man hired to work most of the year after school and full-time during the summer. At one time, Dad used Dean to work for him. Dean remembers that one time he came out to the farm and he saw me swinging on my swing set. Dean is my husband, and he went to school with Gary and played football together. Gary always gave ideas to Dad on whom to hire and I understand that Dad paid real good for the time. But he did hire a young man that I had known all my life, and when we were little, we played together at the lake since our parents were good friends. G.W. changed our lives, and this is the story about him.

G.W. was a year younger than me, and when we were little, he came to my birthday out at the farm.

Dad hired G.W. the end of his sophomore year. He had no experience driving a tractor or working on a farm. He was a fast learner, and by the time he started his junior year of high school, he knew what he was doing, and when Dad would tell him what field or what to do, he just did it. Also, he had bought a car and that was his baby.

I would fix the noon meal during the summer since Mom was working. He always liked leftover days and loved the chocolate chip cookies. If he got in early for lunch, he would help me set the table or anything that needed doing.

At school, we always saw each other and said hello; it was like we were checking on each other, and after school, he would ask if I needed a ride to Mom's office or home. G.W. was thought of highly by his class and was very smart. He was just a good guy.

We would hang out together, and my best friend, Debby, and G.W. were classmates, so the three of us would ride around together in Lindsborg. There was a gas station that was out of business and that was usually where everyone would meet. Then we would drag Main Street and made U-turns, but now I noticed that no more U-turns are allowed on Main Street.

I was chief cook and bottle washer, and I would bring G.W. a sack lunch to the field if he worked late.

I would also bring his car to him at the field, and I had special instructions to follow. I had to let his car idle for five minutes before I drove it. There were a few more instructions, but I can't remember them. He would park the tractor and bring me back home.

He would always wash up in the washroom and then lightly knock on the window in the kitchen door and look in. I remember when I had started dating

Dean and I was getting ready to go out. I had long hair, and to straighten my hair I came up with a way that worked. I washed out four large orange juice cans and bought some long bobby pins, and after the washing, I would put my hair in a ponytail on top of my head and roll my hair on the juice cans, and this seemed to work. There were no large rollers at the time, so I made due. Anyway, when G.W. looked through the window, I scared him enough to where he jumped back about a yard. Dad wondered what he was doing until he saw me but never made a comment, just chuckled.

On my seventeenth birthday, my parents were going to a club that they belonged to, and I was fixing supper for Dean; we had just started dating. Everything was going perfectly until my two-layer chocolate cake fell on one side, and I was so upset. I wanted everything perfect, and I had never had a cake fall and wondered why then. I showed Dad, and I had already frosted the cake before it fell, so all Dad did was take a large knife and cut the part off that fell. G.W. and I couldn't believe what Dad did, but it looked okay, as if someone had cut a couple of pieces out, and Dad and G.W. ate the part Dad cut out with coffee, and G.W. always reminded me of that. He thought that Dad handled it pretty well, but he was glad that he was there when it happened.

Dad bought a brand new pickup truck and let me take it to town to show Debby. Well, we went riding around and saw G.W. So he got in and we drove around for hours without leaving the city limits and put fifty miles on it. Dad wasn't happy with me the next morning when he drove the truck out of the shed. He always thought that we had left the city limits and went to Salina or McPherson, but we didn't.

At the junior-senior prom, Debby and I were dating older guys and didn't bring them. So she and I met our other girlfriends and went as a group. We sat at the stag table, and several other guys sat with us. Some were in the same situation that we were, and G.W. was with them, but he didn't have a date. Looking around, I noticed that everybody else was quiet, and our table had such a good time. After the prom was over, we all ended up on Main Street, and at 1:00 a.m. we were told by the Lindsborg Police to move our cars or they would give us a ticket for loitering. We moved but didn't tell anyone. I went home around 2:00 a.m. because Dean was coming home from college for the weekend. G.W. liked Dean and sure was shocked when we first started dating, and as time went on, he told me that Dean was the one.

After my graduation from high school, my folks had a party at the house and lots of their friends showed up. Dean was right beside me when G.W. showed up and congratulated me; we joked that he was a senior, and the next year I would be congratulating him. I told him that the year would go so fast, and I also invited him to visit Dean and me at Fort Hays Kansas State College.

The summer was big and busy because Dad had taken on more land, and it was the first year for the crops on this land. Nineteen seventy-four was a great year for the farmers. We started irrigating, and this was the second summer, which went a lot better.

Dean and I had been dating almost a year, and we had started talking about marriage. The time came when we left for college. Fall had come, and we went home for break, and it was late October. Dean always went out with his friend to the beer hall on Friday night. So I went to see Debby and catch up on all the gossip. We drove around and went out to B's and got something to drink and then went back up town, and we saw G.W. We stopped and said hi and talked about how were things going. He said that everything was great, and soon after, we were talking, some guys came by and asked G.W. to go someplace. We said our good-byes, and he said he was working at the farm on Saturday.

He worked, but we saw him for lunch and afternoon coffee. Dean and I were sitting outside when he and Dad finished up for the day, and he talked to us while Dad got his weekly paycheck ready. Off he went in his car, and he waved as he drove out the driveway.

We went back to school, and everything was fine. I had spent the night over at Dean's place. It was Sunday morning, and I was fixing a late lunch, and Dean was out dumping the trash when the phone rang and I answered it.

A Day of Unanswered Questions

Dad said hi, but he was surprised to hear my voice, and I told him we were getting ready for lunch, and then I noticed his voice was different. I had never heard his voice like this before. He told me that something horrible had happened, and he wanted me to just listen to what he had to say. Then it came out like a ton of bricks. G.W. was dead. I didn't quite understand what he had just said. G.W. was killed in a car wreck that morning, but there was more to the story, but I started screaming, and Dean came running. He talked with Dad for a while, and his face turned pale white. Dean then hung up the phone and said that he needed to tell me the whole story, and when I calmed down to call Dad back. I felt so sick that I ran to the bathroom, and when I came out, I saw the tears in Dean's eyes. He put his arm around me, and he started telling me what had happened. GW was killed in a one-car accident, and I thought that was strange.

The night before, he had an accident in his car up town, and of course everyone was there. He got the ticket and was upset because his parents had taken the truck to their house at the lake, and it was just him and his brother at the house all night. He must have built himself in such a state about how he was going to explain to his parents that he wrote them a note and took their good car. G.W. ended up hitting a bridge. It was like they were talking about somebody else. This wasn't the G.W. I knew, but I wished he would have called someone. Nobody in their wildest imagination would have thought that he would ever do this horrible thing.

Thursday morning, we went to our advisers to tell them we were going to a funeral and would be back in classes on Friday. We left on Thursday afternoon, and when we got to the farm, my parents met us at the door, and the tears started all over since I hadn't talked to Mom. Dean went on home to his mother's house, and we ate a little supper and were supposed to meet Gary and his wife Linda at the funeral home for the viewing, and I really didn't know if I was ready to say good-bye, but I knew if I didn't do it now, I wouldn't get to. It seemed that everything went into slow motion. I still had my grandparents and really hadn't even been to a lot of funerals.

He had been hurt badly, and as I thought that, Dad said the same thing out loud. I didn't realize how badly Dad hurt. He had been with him a lot, and he really enjoyed having G.W. around. I remember sitting down, and, all of a sudden, I noticed G.W. had his class ring on, and I didn't think he liked it very much, but I was so overwhelmed that I didn't know if that was right or not. He had just had his graduation picture done, and I think he was dressed in the same suit, and then the time had come. Good-bye, friend. I will miss you.

That night, I sat on the end of my bed and was looking out the window where I had sat waiting for Dean so many times. But that night was foggy, and the yard light gave me enough light to see where G.W. used to park his car because it was protected by the trees and the garage. It was like his own driveway. Little did I know my parents didn't sleep much that night, and during the night, we ran in to each other several times, either going to the bathroom, getting something to drink, or taking some Tylenol.

The next morning, we got ready for the funeral,

and I had hoped we weren't going out to the cemetery, and Dean wanted to get back to Hays, so I excused myself and was ready to go right away after the service. I saw Debby, but neither one of us had anything to say at the time, and I couldn't handle seeing his parents. That would come much later.

Dean and I didn't say a lot on the way back, and all I wanted was to be let off at my dorm and needed to be by myself, but Dean returned, and as soon as I saw him, I didn't want him to leave, so we went back to his place, and his roommate was there. I don't remember anything that was said; all I was thinking of was a friend I said good-bye to.

A special thank you to the parents and family of G.W. for allowing me to write about him and remembering all the times we had together. There would have been a chapter missing if he hadn't been in my book. Thank you.

DAD AND THE CATTLE SALES

As I have indicated, we had cattle, that four-legged income. I always tagged along with my father since Gary was at school, and the days that we went to the cattle sales is always a great memory for me.

This is one of my favorite stories, and I hope you enjoy it.

I tagged along with Dad everywhere. If he went to get parts for the equipment, I would go. If he went to town to the Farmers Union to do business or to the bank, I would sit in the lobby, and the secretary to the banker would give me a box of Cracker Jacks, so until she passed on, she was always know as the "Cracker Jack Lady." Dad went to a funeral one time, and of course, he wouldn't take me, and it broke my heart that I couldn't go, or when he was a member of the Lindsborg Lyons Club and on Monday nights, in order to get my mind off him leaving, Mom use to say he was going to roar with the Lyons.

But Tuesdays were our day because I used to love to go to the cattle sales in Salina.

The sale barn was actually a big red barn on the east side of town that smelled of cattle and other things. My favorite memory was what Dad used to wear. He wore a brown corduroy coat and always carried a wood cane. The smell of the coat is still strong in my mind; it smelled like the sale barn, and he would smoke a cigar while looking at or watching what his cattle would bring. That was a great coat.

We sat on wooden bleachers, and I suppose the building was heated, but Mom always dressed me in warm clothes, and I always brought a jacket for the brisk evening when we were going home. Sitting by Dad was so exciting, watching him bid, and the auctioneer always shocked me with how he could talk so fast.

The first thing Dad taught me was to never hold your hand up or scratch your nose when the auctioneer was talking. He said that I could scratch or move my hand around in between the bids or sit on them if I had to. Dad never seemed bothered about taking me with him, and the men always tried to flirt with me, and I would hide behind my dad's coat and feel safe.

If he bought cattle, there was always lots of paperwork to do. First was to arrange transportation for the cattle home, and he used this one man all the time. Then Dad got the paperwork to the driver so he would know what cattle were going home with us, and with all the times he had been to our farm, he was like an old friend. Then the best part of the whole day was going to the restaurant where the waitress always knew what we ordered. Dad ordered me a piece of homemade chocolate pie and a bottle of grape pop. Dad always had his favorite, homemade lemon meringue pie with coffee. I always enjoyed watching the people, and I saw the trucker having a huge dinner because he knew it was going to be a long night.

There weren't any cattle sales during the summer because all the farmers were working in the fields and baling hay and preparing for the fall and winter months, so it was usually very cold by evening when we started for home.

We always were in the truck. After eating a big piece of pie and drinking a pop, I was full, and when Dad put the heater on in the truck, it didn't take any time for me to get sleepy. I would lay my head down on Dad's lap, and he would put the corduroy coat over me, and in no time we were pulling in the driveway, and the semi was usually behind us. Dad let me off at the house and usually Gary was on his way out to the loading shoot and when Mom saw me she always laughed because Dad never washed my face, and I had a grape pop and chocolate pie mustache.

We would always walk out to the corral and see our new residents. Gary had already gotten the feed out and made sure there was lots of hay ready for supper. The fresh water had been run from the well. The driver always helped unload, and this is when Dad used the cane to poke the cattle's bottoms so they wouldn't fall down and get trampled. The cane kept them going at a nice, safe pace. When they were settled and the trucker had been paid and left, we had our supper. With all the excitement, we were ready for bed, and since Gary's and my room faced the east, we heard the cattle bawl all night because they were scared and didn't know where they were. Sometimes Dad would come in with that cow poop smell, and he always said it was the smell of money.

Later on, when we were older and in school, Dad would let us have a calf, and he would mark it for us.

We would move them closer and feed them, and they actually became our pets. Dad always decided when the cows were big enough, he would sell them for us, and there would be a check in both our names that we signed, and he put them in our savings account. He always said he took a percentage out for feed and hay. But I always wondered if he did.

A Special Day

It was in October of '73, and it was my senior year in high school. Dad was going to the cattle sale and wanted to know if I wanted to go with him. He knew that I was dating Dean and that he was probably the one that I would marry in the future and that I was off to college in a year. So he called the school and took one of my senior days, and he pulled the truck up to the house, and away we went.

When we got to Salina, we turned the wrong way, and then I found out that the red barn had burned down a few years ago, and there was a new barn on the northwest side of Salina. It was a huge building, and there was an office where the farmers and ranchers were able to sit down and do the paperwork, and there was a real nice restaurant. We walked in to the sales part of the building, and there were no wooden benches but actual metal seats, but I thought that the wooden benches were more comfortable. The auctioneer and the guys that worked in the arena were the same men, but they were a little older, and some of the audience that I knew was showing their age. There was a woman sitting with her husband, cross-stitching. I always enjoyed watching them, especially when they would send a bull out and then he got wild.

All the men that used to scare me before talked to me and I talked back now. I enjoyed seeing those guys again, but I think that Dad was glad that we went to the cattle sale because it was the last one.

We did our same routine and finally went into the restaurant, and Dad ordered his usual, but the waitress had his order down, and when she asked what I wanted, I looked at her, and she couldn't believe her eyes. She then asked if I wanted my usual. I said homemade chocolate pie and an iced tea. She acted let down when I said iced tea instead of grape pop, but she understood. We enjoyed the day. I wasn't tired when we headed for home, but I asked Dad if I could wear his brown corduroy coat, and he put it around my shoulder. The smell was still there, the one that was there when I was his little girl.

The last time I saw the coat was at the house they moved to from the farm. It was hanging on a hook in the basement stairwell, like out at the farm, and the smell was still there, but it wasn't as pungent as it used to be, and Dad gave the cane to me when I was having trouble with my muscles after the withdrawal, and it is still hanging on my coat rack, and I always know where it's at. One time, I had the girls smell the coat, and they said it smelled like Grandpa. They had been told the story many times at bedtime.

KANOPOLIS STATE LAKE

Mom and Dad started going to the lake when they first came back to Lindsborg. The lake is only a fifteen-minute drive from the farmhouse. They enjoyed meeting their friends and families after church during the summer.

There were nice beaches, and many sand castles were built on those beaches. We had a lot of fun; in fact, this is where I met GW and Lisa, playing on the beach. There were so many kids between Gary and I, we never ran out of friends. Eventually, some of the parents bought boats and would ask us to go for a ride around the lake, which was large to me. I really liked that part of the day and watching the water skiers. There was a large building that you walked through, and it had a concession stand, but Mom always brought treats and jugs of icy cold lemonade and iced tea. I remember that Mom always had to have a lot of ice for her tea and that it used to bug Dad, but I am the same way, and he knows where I got that from.

Anyway, when it was time to head home, we always looked along the Smoky Hill River to see if there were any deer around the edge. Then we always would sing, and one song, "I Drove a Herd of Cattle," was one of our favorites.

Before Dad could move into his apartment, there was a month that he came to stay with us. He and I used to watch the Western channel together at lunch, and suddenly we heard that song. The *Gene Autry Show* was on, and he was singing the song. Dad and I looked at each other in shock and laughed.

Eventually, Dad and Mom bought a boat, which was great. When we were on the dock, we would always load things and take a trip around the lake. We would then meet up with the group, which had now found a real nice place to be. Families were now camping in their tents. Everyone brought their own barbecues and would end up eating an early supper before we left. I don't ever remember eating a hot dog or hamburger without a dash of sand.

Dad, Mom, and Gary soon learned to water ski, and Dad gave us signals to watch for by the skier in case the skier was tired or something else. I didn't learn to water ski for a long time. I wasn't afraid; I just couldn't get up. We tried children's skis and that didn't work, so I always rode along watching for Dad as he drove the boat. I remember Mom waving at me, and Gary would make faces at me. What fun.

We went on vacation to the Lake of the Ozarks and stayed at a lodge called Shangri La. Dad was going over across the lake to buy gas for the boat. We were along for a ride, and I asked if I could try skiing again. All we had were the adult skis, so Gary made the feet as small as it would go. I was ready to go, and I gave a wave of my hand, and away we went. I got right up on skis for adults, and I saw three shocked faces in the boat looking at me. Dad couldn't shake me off. I was having so much fun jumping over the waves, and now I was waving at them. I was so exhausted but happy. One time, I fell down and somehow got the rope wrapped around my legs and that hurt.

Gary was the daredevil; he was always trying to outdo himself. He always wanted to try to ski off the dock. He sat down and made sure everything was ready. Dad knew that he was going to speed the boat up. His bottom slipped off the dock, and he was up. We cheered for him until he went back down, he didn't fall either. He had done the trick perfectly until he turned around. He had splinters on his backside, and you should have seen his face when Mom started picking them out. She had to finish at home and that was a rough ride home. The dock was pretreated wood, so the splinters really hurt.

His next trick was that he wanted Dad to drop him off closer so he could ski right up on shore. He hit his mark that he thought he needed with good speed. Once he hit the beach, that's all she wrote. His skies flew off in each direction, and he went flying through the air, landing face first in the sand. Come to think of it, that would have been a great video for *America's Funniest Home Videos.* You should have seen his ski tracks start up the beach and just stop.

I couldn't even begin to count the people we taught to ski. We finally got a larger boat with a larger motor. Dad could pull two skiers at a time. He would push the throttle down and away you went, almost pulled out of your skis.

Once in a while, when it wasn't as busy, Dad would let us dive off the boat in the middle of the lake. We had our life jackets on. We would climb back in and see who could do the stupidest dives. We will always remember the time we loaded the boat and started off. Water was coming in, and we started bailing out water. All of a sudden Dad remembered he had forgotten to put the plug in. So we hurried back to land, unloaded the boat, and put the plug in. Close call.

Sundays were lots of fun, but during the week, if there had been rain or a thunderstorm, all the farm work came to a stop. We would do a few chores, and we had our own jobs to do to get ready to go. All you would have to say was "Lake, anybody?" and we could be on the road in fifteen minutes. Going during the week was always great because we usually had the beach to ourselves, and the water had no white caps. You haven't skied on water until you ski on water that looks like glass. Your skis would make this sound, like skimming over the water, barely touching the water. The spray from the back of your skis would shine, and you could almost see a rainbow, as if the water was a prism.

The lake is still a beautiful sight today. Some things have changed, including all the new cabins and places for the campers and motor homes that you can rent. Parks have been put in for the kids to play, and there are basketball courts and volleyball nets. You know, that old saying, "The family that works together plays together."

THE DAYS OF WINTER

On the snowy days, we just didn't sit around in the house; we were outside sledding. We had several good hills around our house, and it was always hard to decide where we wanted to go.

Sometimes Dad would tie a long rope on our sled and take us for a ride in back of the tractor. The pasture was a great place for this kind of sledding. Gary sat in front, and I sat on the back, holding on for dear life. We laughed because Gary maneuvered the sled with his feet. Of course, we would fall off the sled, and it wasn't very far to the ground, where we usually ended up with a face full of snow.

On Christmas Day, we found a two-seater sled under the tree from Santa. We went to the bigger hill just to the north of our house. We went down so fast, which was great fun, but climbing back up the hill took forever. Mom and Dad even tried out our new sled and took many rides that we didn't know when we would get our sled back. My parents should have asked Santa for a sled too.

Ice Skating with the Bengtsons

Our neighbors were the Bengtsons. Dad and Gilbert had grown up together, and both were farmers. Irene and Mom gave each other perms. Do you remember the Toni home perms? We took vacations with the Bengston's but I remember I felt left out because they had all boys. We would go to their pond south of their house and go ice skating. No ice skates needed, just our rubber snow boots. Mom always put bread bags between our shoes and the boots so our feet didn't get wet. Dad and Gilbert made a fire, and Mom and Irene had brought hot chocolate and coffee for them, and cookies, of course. The boys rode their bikes; racing on the ice got pretty wild. I remember the roasted marshmallows and making s'mores.

Our parents brought their lawn chairs and pulled logs up for us kids to sit on. The boys would try all kinds of stupid stuff on the ice. They would fall off their bikes and slide across the pond.

A lot of times, I would lay on my Dad's lap and be so warm by the fire and would go off to sleep but would wake up when they decided to let the fire go out. That's when they made the boys stand by the fire to dry off before they got back in the truck. You never want to forget those evenings. Gilbert is gone, but I bet if you ask Irene, John, and Don, they would remember those evenings.

Gary had a wild idea to cut a car's hood off and go sledding. He thought that the hood would spin; it did, and we flew out. Dad said that it looked too dangerous, so Gary had to get rid of it, but not until several of his friends got to try it. What fun.

Many years before, Grandpa had put the old sleigh and horse buggy up in the hayloft. They actually used them to go to town in, depending on the season. We had such a great time playing in the buggy and the sleigh that our imagination just took off.

The Present

The following Christmas Eve, Gary carried in a huge present wrapped in black trash bags. He set it down by me, and I remember everyone telling me to open it. As everyone got quiet, I opened up the gift. It was the old bench from the sled, but Gary had built a box to go under the bench, and Linda finished it up with a heritage blue and painted a Swedish design on the seat. They finished the project off with black rod iron to hold the seat together. In fact, as I am writing this story, I am sitting and looking right at the bench. This is probably the best gift that I have ever gotten for Christmas. Gary got the other seat for himself. My grandparents actually used the sleigh to go to church and blankets to keep warm. They would tie the horses to the hitching post in front of the church.

But this Christmas was the first holiday in my parents' new house in Lindsborg, and it had been five months since we lost our little girl, Stacy. Gary's gift couldn't have come at a better time. I came to realize that we wouldn't be going home anymore but to visit our parents at the home.

I always look at that seat and remember the fun that Gary and I once had, playing up in the hayloft.

TORNADO

In 1973, September was still a little warm, but it seemed that tornado season was over for the year. Well, Mother Nature sure had something to say about that subject.

Mom and Dad were watching the evening news and were talking over the day they had had. This was their routine in the evenings, and we always had supper after the news.

Grandma called, and I picked up the phone that was in my parents' room. The sirens were going off in Lindsborg, indicating that there was a tornado sighting to the southwest of us. While listening to her, I just happened to roll the shade up on the window that looked out to the west. There was a huge cloud hanging over the hills, and it looked kind of strange. All of a sudden, I spotted the tornado and told Grandma that I saw it and hung up on her.

I started down the stairs, which seemed to take forever, like in slow motion. Mom and Dad had just seen the warning on the TV, and I yelled that I had seen the tornado. I thought that it was interesting how Dad commented on how clear the picture was on the TV. It has been said that when the picture was clear, a tornado was around. We had just an antenna.

We ran outside, and once out in the yard, there it was. At first it looked like a rope, and then the most unlikely thing happened. My parents stood in the yard while the tornado was roaring down the hill, swinging its tail as if it were mad, and argued loudly where they should go for shelter. There were two places, but they couldn't make up their minds.

We always thought that down the basement and under an old table was the best place, but Dad was worried that the house would come down on top of us. He thought that we should go to the old cave they had once used for meat and to keep things cool. Mom didn't want to go there because of all the creepy critters, spiders, and possibly a snake.

Now, at this point in time, our cousins lived across the road from us and were in the path of the tornado.

Melvin was busy with his movie camera, and Emma was already in the shelter, yelling for him to come. I, on the other hand, thought my parents were nuts, but I remember how calm it was with a roar in the background. Then suddenly the tornado made a change in direction and went around our cousins' house and was twilling around in the pasture across from our house. It was a tremendous feeling watching this funnel that had grown bigger all of a sudden. It moved on, staying on the other side of the road, and my parents got real quiet. It had left, and where did it go? We got in the car, which you never do in a tornado, and as we reached the end of the driveway, we saw Gilbert, Irene, and Don in their pickup following after the storm.

So they followed us, and all of a sudden you could see that it had eaten something. So about two miles on down the road, we had to stop because of all the poles, tree limbs, and lots of lines that had been pulled down. Gilbert was worried about his brother's house, so we all walked in.

It had hit the outbuildings in the barnyard but missed his brother's house and jumped the road to the farm across the road. What a mess. The tornado had really done a job and rolled off in a northeastern path.

The house had been moved about eight inches off its foundation, and all the items that were in the windows were all standing in their places as if nothing had happened. There had been a combine that was picked up and slammed into the ground and looked like toothpicks all over. The side of the house was plastered with mud. A few outbuildings, such as the barns, had really taken a beating. The funniest thing I saw was the outhouse turned upside down. The two-seater was now a toilet with seats that hung from the ceiling and the door swung the other way. Tornadoes sometimes have a strange sense of humor.

No one had gotten hurt, and the damage was minimal, but I still couldn't understand my parents. We got to see the film that Melvin took and that's when it dawned on me that Mother Nature just didn't want to be involved in the argument that my parents were having, and you could see on the film the way it switched directions.

There was a lot of rain that followed along the back of the tornado, but that didn't stop people from checking on us. Dean said that it looked like the tornado had hit our house. He was worried what he would find. Gary had the same feeling.

When nightfall came, there wasn't a breath of wind, as if the whole agonizing ordeal had never happened. The rainbows were really bright, and the sunset was one of the prettiest I had ever seen.

The ending of this story is that I don't think that my parents ever decided where to go the next time, but everything ended up great, because the next year at college, I took a writing class, and this was the first story I had written, and I got an A.

SOMETHING WAS WRONG

A short time after moving back to Lindsborg, my gallbladder had been causing me problems, and when we got moved in and everyone was settled, I had an attack and couldn't handle the pain, so Dean took me to the hospital, and I had my gallbladder removed. I didn't have it easy; they had to make a long incision. I haven't regretted losing it, but I had an infection for a while afterward. Once that cleared up, I felt okay, but I felt that something else was wrong.

Months later, I started having breathing problems, and then the breathing attacks came on. My family physician (FP) decided he wanted a second opinion, and I was okay with that. So I ended up seeing a pulmonary doctor. When I started seeing him, he ran no tests, no blood tests, and no X-rays but said I had asthma due to allergies. An hour later, Dean and I were walking out of his office with samples of inhalers and a prescription for a machine to do treatments with four times a day. This is where I started taking steroids and gained some weight. I read the instructions to the machine, and it reminded me of a machine you use at the hospital to clear your lungs out. Taking all the medicines used up a good portion of my day.

I had routine appointments with the pulmonary doctor; Dean asked him why I was weak, and his answer was because it took time to get the right combination of medicine. By this time, I was on a lot of prescription medication. I was having good days and bad days but started having to go to the hospital more and more because I still couldn't breath. Then they started keeping me overnight, and then I really started hating life. I don't ever remember feeling stable, and I had a nagging feeling that we were missing something. I wondered if maybe I wasn't taking the medicine right, so I wrote down my medications and when I took them and carried it with me wherever I went. Then my blood pressure started going up; it was dangerously high, and they started me on blood pressure medicine, and I felt better. I thought the headaches were from not breathing well, but it was the blood pressure causing that problem. By this time, my system was very touchy with medications.

I felt like I was held captive in my own home. Because of not feeling well, I didn't have any energy to go anywhere, and by the time I got dressed and ready to go, I was exhausted. At this time, it was affecting my family, all the time I missed with my husband and girls and the things I missed and never got back.

My family also saw a change in me that scared them. Mom and Dad would come over and bring casseroles for supper, and they checked on me frequently. All I could do was wash out the pans and send them back for the next week. The stress was building up in me, and that didn't help anything—breathing, blood pressure, or even my mental abilities.

I would try to hold down part-time jobs because I thought this would get me out of the house. But I failed at most of them. Failed is a horrible word to use, but I tried.

Also at this time, we noticed that when Mom would stand up, she would lose her balance and fall down. The doctors told her that when she stood up, her blood pressure would sink. They wanted her to stand in one place for a minute or two and then walk. It didn't happen all the time, but when she would fall, she always knew what happened, and everyone would just help her up.

Most of the time, I felt like I was high and felt like I was walking in slow motion. My memory wasn't good, so my girls bought me a notebook to write things in, and in that notebook, nothing made sense; my writing had changed; my whole personality changed; something was really wrong, but I couldn't explain it.

At my appointments, the pulmonary doctor always kept telling Dean that we had just not found the right combination, and my parents feared that with all the prescriptions, eventually I was going to take the wrong combination, and they wouldn't have me anymore. Dean thought the same way but had too much on his plate at the time. My family was coming apart at the seams, and there was nothing I could do.

The depression set in, but I refused any more medications, which was stupid; that's the medication I should have been taking. My thinking wasn't exactly straight. My FP didn't know what to do with me.

But everybody, from the hospital to the doctors, stuck in with me.

One day, Dean got mad when I had another appointment with the pulmonary doctor, and he wanted an explanation for the personality changes, and he also talked about other people with asthma not having the problems that I was having. He actually told him that I was walking around and looked like "death warmed over." The physician always had answers, and we would leave his office feeling better than we did going in. Yet my symptoms were not going away. The mental and physical changes really were starting to scare me, and I knew if something didn't change soon, I was going to be in trouble.

The Nightmare Begins

In February of 1994, my life was on a continuous roller coaster, and when I got up in the morning, I never knew if I would be sleeping in the hospital that night, and my whole family was on this roller coaster ride with me. Although I didn't know it, I was hooked on prescription drugs. Even though I was seeing a doctor, my life was horrible, but I still hung in. By now I was working part-time again and not being successful at that. My mom and I had plans to attend the mother-daughter banquet, and I even had bought a new outfit for the occasion.

The day started off badly because I had been up most the night having trouble breathing again. I took an extra treatment, and I started shaking from the medication and hoped by daylight I could back off a treatment, but that wasn't going to happen. In my mind, I thought that I wasn't going to be able to work that afternoon, and I knew I was on the edge of being fired then. Then Mom bought the tickets that evening. The banquet was held at the church, and it was fun to see the men from the congregation wearing aprons and serving the women. They always had a show after dinner, and Mom and I always looked forward to the mother-daughter banquet. These things were not helping.

The phone rang, and I didn't even have to look at the caller ID to know it was Mom. We called each other every morning after I got the girls off to school. She knew right away something was wrong but didn't comment too much. Mom would always make sure, that even though we had become adults. That she was still our mom, and usually what she said, goes. But she knew she was taking a big chance. She always could tell by the sound of our voices, something was wrong. If you tried to hide your problem, she would be knocking at your door.

When we got to the ER, my fingernails and the area around my mouth was blue, my blood pressure was extremely high, and they called the doctor to the room ASAP. Things got really hazy until a nurse came in and stuck a needle in my wrist for blood to find out how much oxygen was in my blood. I remember feeling really bad, and the nurse asked my mom to step out of the room, and then everything went blank.

When I woke up, Mom was beside me, holding my hand, and I remember she was shaking. Her blue eyes were really bright, and I knew she had been crying. She told me that I was stable, and they were moving me to a room in a little while, so she was going to get Dean and Dad, check in on the girls, and make a couple of phone calls. She told me she would be back and not to go anywhere and that she loved me very much. I then looked around a little better because my eyesight cleared up. I had oxygen and an IV going, and a machine was taking my blood pressure every ten minutes, and I realized something really had gone wrong. But I was too tired to worry about it, and all I wanted to do was sleep. I remember waking up and wondering where Mom was but just didn't have the energy to ask.

Mom went to the college to find Dean and went to his office, and he was just getting ready to come home. He said that Mom had a look that he would never forget. She told him what happened and where I was and what the doctor said, and all he heard was life- threatening asthma and the attack had been real bad. Dean told her to go to the house for the girls, and he was on the way to see me. He didn't want the girls to come to the hospital until I had improved. I woke up and he was holding my hand, and I then knew everything was going to be okay.

After a couple of days in the hospital, I had gained my strength back and was ready to go home. Everything was looking up, except the medicines had been changed and a shot of Depo-Medrol once a week, which was another steroid, and the doctor ordered the shot to be given in Lindsborg.

But it finally was a nurse that told me what happened; I had almost died. Dean had known, but it was a shock to me. Then I knew I wanted out of the hospital and to go home as soon as possible. The doctor was in the middle of his rounds, and once he got to my room, the mood changed. He explained the changes in the medicine and about the shots and said to stay home from work until he saw me in two weeks.

When I got home, laying on the table was something that had been from the Mother/ Daughter banquet and I found out that one of my girls had gone with mom. I was so proud. I was feeling better, but something was still nagging me.

Time Would Tell

I got my first shot a week after I left the hospital, and Dean took me to my follow-up appointment, and I asked exactly what was in the shot. I found out there was Depo-Medrol. Depo-Medrol is another steroid that is stronger, but I couldn't figure out why I was taking two different types of steroids, but I didn't ask any questions because I trusted my pulmonary doctor. Then, we couldn't believe what he said next. He said he wasn't sure he could save me, if I had another attack. We were shocked at the way he said it, like he was covering something up. The new list of medicine was long, but I was back at work in no time.

Months went on and I had a couple of attacks, but nothing like that big one. But that nagging feeling was getting stronger and really started to bother me to where I couldn't shake it. After a couple more visits with the pulmonary doctor, I got uneasy feeling that he really didn't care any more. Dean thought that he couldn't do anymore for me, so why try, like I wasn't good enough to be in his presence. After that appointment, I never went back. It was time to follow that feeling, but how was I going to get the doctors to believe me?

I went back to where we started from, our FD, and I told the PA how I felt, and he talked to one of the doctors to discuss what could be done. They told me of a place that was out of state and they could probably diagnose the problem and I was for that, and my insurance company went along with me. The only thing stopping us was that they wanted me to go through withdrawal before I got there. They told the doctors to make a plan and that they would be a phone call away if the attacks came back on.

The plan was to not take my next shot and to go slowly off all the other medications except my blood pressure medicine. Then when the symptoms worsened, I would enter the hospital for IVs , oxygen, and whatever else they could do to support me. No pain medications except Tylenol. We had a few days to decide, and we had a family meeting about the plan.

Finally, everyone was in agreement. The next item on the list was quitting my job. I think everyone felt that I had a good reason.

I knew that this was one of the hardest problems that I would have, at least in the top five on my list. One more thing is that I wrote and signed a piece of paper to only administer drugs for a life-threatening problem, and so it begins…

WITHDRAWAL, HERE I GO

Within a week, the side effects showed their ugly face, but that was nothing compared to what was going to happen. At first, the headaches were strong, and they had me drinking a two-liter bottle of water, but I thought it was more like a blood pressure problem, and Tylenol didn't help. Then, ten days later, I had an appointment at the doctor's office, but I had already been vomiting and I was already dehydrated, and my blood pressure was high. So they decided it was time to enter the hospital and get the IVs started so they could administer blood pressure medicine through the IVs . Then they ordered a wheelchair to go over to the hospital, and I said no; I was walking in on my own, and I'd be walking out on my own. So I walked between Dean and the PA; they were watching me because I had that blue tint around my mouth. So once I was settled, they put oxygen on.

The next day, I didn't want any company, and I laid in one position because it felt like I had been hit by a MAC truck. By evening, the shaking started and I vomited white foam. Mom and Dad were there, and Mom was rubbing my head like she used to do when I was a kid. It felt great; her hands were warm, and I was so cold. From there on, it was hell, but somehow God let me forget most of it. Mom said they wrapped the bed and headboard with towels because I shook so hard and the bed was hitting the wall. I guess that the hospital bed just rattled. I looked like a fright that Dean decided the girls couldn't see me until this part was over.

Either Mom and Dad were up at the hospital every morning, hoping that there was better news than what they were seeing. Dean couldn't stand to see me like this. He checked on me every day but didn't sit and watch. He would always be there when the doctors did their rounds; they kept saying that everything was going to the plan. The nurses were still watching me, taking my blood pressure and mainly just watching. Days went on until I started coming around. I was so exhausted and I hurt everywhere. But I started looking at people and knew who they were.

Finally, I remember my Dad standing over by the window, watching the helicopter landing for a patient. I remember saying hi, and he looked around and just stared at me. He then came over to the bed and leaned over and said "Hi, Tootsie." We didn't talk much, and by the time he rang for a nurse, I was back to sleep again, but now I heard everyone talking, and I understood what they were saying. Mom was there the next time I woke up, and she had decided to be there if it took all day. I said hi and she cried. They came in, took my blood, and then the doctor would ask me some questions, and I got lost. Dean was concerned, but the doctor said the more rest I got, the more everything would come back, and if that didn't happen, they would get me help. Dean was there with me, and I knew everything was going to be okay. My blood pressure and pulse were better but not stable yet, and I knew they were watching something with my blood.

The girls got to visit me a couple days later, and I wanted to catch up on what they were doing. Angie had tried out for cheerleading in the seventh and eighth grade and got a place on the team. The first football game was in two weeks, and she needed a few things, so Jennifer took her shopping, and when she got her uniform, she brought it up to show me. Jennifer had a job and a boyfriend that Dean didn't like and that put a wedge between them and that wedge was still there; you could feel it when they all came to visit me.

My oxygen levels and my blood pressure were returning back to normal, and we thought it was strange how there had been no asthma attacks, none. So they started letting me get out of bed and sitting in the chairs. The only thing was I couldn't read and keep my mind on the book, so a nurse that was on the night shift started me on counted cross-stitch, and then I remembered that another friend had started me on it before. I was still shaking a lot, and every stitch was a stitch more than the day before. The night nurse would check it and brought in some supplies for me.

The doctors decided to start me on Tylenol every four hours for the pain. They finally let me take a shower, and I was sweating so much that they turned the air conditioning up and put a fan in the room. When someone came to visit, he or she brought a sweater or jacket. The nurses commented that I had really went through an ordeal.

By the way, the picture that I cross-stitched, I finished and had it framed. It was a Christmas gift for my parents the following year. They knew how hard I worked on it and the shaking I did. They really liked it and hung it in their hallway. I was proud too.

The lab was still taking lots of blood every other day at 4:00 p.m. I still felt there was something not right with my body. I was always so tired in the afternoon and usually slept all afternoon. There were days that I would never want to live through again.

The News

I knew the day when one of the doctors came in that he wasn't bringing me good news. I read his face and just wanted to know what was wrong. He was looking at my chart, and he looked up at me. Then it came: my adrenal glands were failing, and it was almost time to take some recourse.

Your adrenal glands are two triangular-shaped glands located above each kidney. The glands are responsible for controlling lots of functions, including the regulation of salt and water balances in the body. They're also partly responsible for controlling the blood pressure.

My thought was, *Okay, now what do we do to control the problem?* The answer just astonished me and was one I had to think about—one word that I never wanted to hear: steroids.

I started to cry and scream. I couldn't understand. I had gone through the roughest part of the withdrawal and things still weren't good, but I did it, and now they were telling me that I had to go back on the steroids to live a fairly normal life, Prednisone, to be exact, and this wasn't the news that I wanted to hear. I thought that I was ready for anything except this; I felt my strength being sucked out of my body. The hospital staff knew that there wasn't anything else that they could add and just left me alone. I didn't understand anything, and I thought that we would wait and see what the next test would say. The test results were due in the morning, Saturday morning.

The next morning, the nurses brought me some books from their medical library about the endocrine system, and this is what I learned.

Before I go on with the paragraph, this is one of the points of writing this book. When our children take our (their parents) medicine to get a high with, this can happen to them, the withdrawal, the malfunction of the adrenal glands, permanent damage to their heart, and they would be living a lot longer than I am with the problems, especially having the adrenal storms and really don't even know your body. If some kid would take my medication, it won't hurt me. I can always get more medication; they could die. This is really scary.

Your Endocrine System 101

The endocrine system keeps a lot of our bodily functions going. It is a network of glands that produces and secretes hormones involved in controlling many functions of the body. This includes growth and development, stability of internal bodily systems (homeostasis), metabolism, and sexual functions.

The glands that are affected are the pituitary glands, the hypothalamus, the adrenal glands, and the pancreas. I was told that I would have to go back on steroids, the Prednisone, in order to keep my body functioning. But I couldn't go home until my steroid count was back to five. Jennifer had come to visit, and while we were talking, the nurse came in with my results, and I was at a zero. All I could do was cry, and Jennifer just held me and said everything was going to be okay. I couldn't take a chance on catching the flu, cold, or an infection. I was angry. What I didn't think of was what caused my adrenal gland to stop functioning, and I get the answer in the very near future. I would just have to wait. This looked pretty hopeless, but I was glad I didn't know what was next.

REHABILITATION

I looked up rehabilitation in the dictionary: (1) to restore to rank, replace, reputation, etc. which one has lost; (2) to put back in good condition; (3) to bring or restore to a state of health, constructive activity. This pretty much tells the way it is, but they forgot one tiny word. My meaning for rehabilitation was help!

When I was dismissed from the hospital, I was feeling okay, and I did walk out of the hospital on my own with the help of a quad cane. But getting home was an eye-opener. But Mom knew that I would be in the house, and we drove around, getting fresh air, and not being poked really had its pluses. I was a lot weaker than I thought, and the muscular pain wasn't any better and the leg cramps were horrendous.

I noticed that my body as I knew it wasn't the same and that took a lot of time. The exhaustion was so bad that I felt like my arms were dragging on the floor behind me. I was actually getting tired with life and the way it was.

I thought that when I got home that I would get back in a routine of laundry, cooking, and cleaning, but every time I moved, the pain was in different places. I could have just given up and gone to bed and stayed there. That would have been easy. I found out that the recliner in the living room really helped; hot showers and the heating pad were my best friends. I was able to read and understand what I was reading, but the television just brought on the anxiety. Dad came over and we played cards, and then I got interested in puzzles. Dean put up our card table and two chairs in front of the south windows in the living room, and the south rays felt so good in the mornings that I usually was able to sit and work on puzzles all morning. The shakes weren't all the way gone, and some days they were worse. The first appointment back to the doctor was for a blood test, and Dean and I were talking to the PA. He said that he couldn't imagine how I felt, and I thought that was a line of bull. Then he told us a story about when he had gotten mixed up in some poison ivy and had a real bad reaction; they gave him a shot of Depo-Medrol to dry up the rash and the reaction to the ivy, and it helped, but he then had another one two weeks later. The poison ivy went away, but the muscular effects that it had on his body were unbelievable. He couldn't imagine what I had been and was still going through. My doctors were going to see me every two weeks, but it was going to be at least a month before discussing my traveling plan to the out-of-state hospital.

I would say that September was the worst month there had ever been. On top of feeling bad, my parents' goddaughter, Lisa, was killed in an airline disaster. It happened in the evening because I had gotten to go watch Angie cheer at the football game, but we came home at halftime, and Dean turned on the television and we saw about the accident, never thinking that we knew someone on that plane over Pittsburgh. I had to go to the memorial service; I couldn't bear sitting at home. We had grown up together, and it hit my parents hard. Dad helped by picking me up and getting me into the church. I wanted to sit in the back and went home after the service, but I knew I wanted to bring something to her parents since they were like my second parents. All by myself, I bought a turkey and drove out to their home in the country and had a short visit. The best thing is that I did it without help, but I was really exhausted. Dean never knew, but my parents found out later and had a fit.

> In Memory.
>
> To Lisa, my parents' goddaughter. You are so missed, and I was thinking that this year you would be turning fifty years old. I want to thank your parents and the family for letting me put you in the book.
>
> Thank you to my second parents.
>
> Love, Wendy

The time had come when the doctors said it was time to go. A friend was going with me, but we found out that I was staying in the hospital until the testing was done, and I figured that since I was out of town, I would stay there.

Another problem was that I couldn't shake another feeling that I would probably die there, and I kept that thought to myself. The day before I left, we had my parents over, and I said good-bye, which was terrible because I thought I knew something they didn't know, and the next morning when I was packed and ready to go say good-bye to my girls; it was unimaginable. They walked out to the car with Dean and me, and as we pulled away, I remember looking at them through the mirror on the car, thinking that they would be okay and would become young women and have their own lives. I wanted to write a note to Dean and leave it where the girls wouldn't see it, but I just couldn't explain, and I knew he would have been on the first plane to be with me. I was also scared of the airline because it hadn't been long since Lisa had died, but I agonized over how when she walked on to the plane, she had no idea that she wouldn't be getting off. Saying good-bye to Dean was about as horrible as it could get, and they transferred me on the plane by wheelchair, and the pilot happened to be standing there and helped me get seated and made sure that I was safe. He was a real nice guy, and I was impressed that he took the time because that wasn't his job. The flight was really rough on me, but the hospital personnel were at the gate when we landed and got me to the hospital in nothing flat.

I went to the lab and gave a lot of blood; then they took me to my room where my luggage finally caught up to me. All the doctors who were assigned to my case came in and introduced themselves to me, and my attendant brought in my schedule for tests through the week, and it looked like Thursday was a big day for the tests. Friday, the schedule said conference late that afternoon. They left me alone to rest, and I would get ready for the next day of tests.

The tests weren't too bad, and everyone told me that whatever they did, I would be able to walk or ride out. After the first test was over, they took me out to the waiting room. There was a lady looking at a magazine. We didn't say much to each other, and then they took her in and I went to my next appointment. The next days were about the same, but I started going to physical therapy, and that was painful because the more they worked with my legs, the more the cramps came on.

Finally, the last day of tests were done. It was a CT scan and some other X-rays, then the most interesting test of all. They stuck a tube down me and made me do a lot of talking and sounding out vowels, A, E, I, O, and U. I watched my vocal cords move on the TV, and I remember how impressed I was. It wasn't painful, and watching my own vocal cords was kind of neat.

When I went to my meeting, the room was set up as a boardroom with a long table with many chairs.

He started telling me about my body, and of course we already knew about my adrenal gland and the endocrine system and the dose of Prednisone that I should be on, and then he explained what had happened to me, and I noticed that the atmosphere changed.

What had happened was with my gall bladder surgery, when they ventilated me, the tube was probably the wrong size, or it affected me somehow. Then my vocal cords ended up very irritated, and they started working backward and never corrected themselves. They call it vocal cord dysfunction, which tends to act like asthma because the vocal cords rub against each other and swell, causing me not to get much air. This could have been detected with a scope and a CT scan.

Then came the shocking news. I didn't need all the medications or the shots; all this medicine was what blew my adrenal glands. They never said anything about whose fault it was, and anyway it was too late.

This really shattered me.

The next subject was what they could do for me: work with my vocal cords, physical therapy, and occupational therapy. They asked me if I brought my swimming suit like they told me to in the brochure. The handicap pool was eighty degrees, and they had bars to hang on to, and with the water buoyancy, the physical therapy would help me move easier in the water and could help the spasms. Then I had to learn to walk with the cane the right way, and they had me walking all over the hallways and then learning to walk up the stairs. No more wheelchair; it was time to get my body back in shape, and it was mind over matter.

Then I had to work on healing the mind, so I started visiting with a psychologist. After I went back to my room and remembered all that was said and cried, I called my soul mate, Dean, and told him everything that was said in the meeting, and I could hear the anger in his voice. When he calmed down and I stopped crying, I told him that I was going to be walking off the plane and into his arms.

There was a knock on my door, and a younger woman walked in and introduced herself as the psychologist and thought that I needed to talk. She told me she was glad to see me crying because crying was the first step to recovery. I thought she was nuts, and she was the doctor! As we started to talk, it was if she had known me all my life. But this was from all the paperwork that my doctors had sent, and she had done her studying already, so she made it very easy. We were together for about two hours, the first session of many. I was exhausted; it had been a long day. A lot of things were thrown at me, and I had to think things through on what I had learned that day. I think that the one thing that just astounded me was overhearing a conversation that I wasn't supposed to hear, but I'm glad I did. It was said by one of the doctors at the meeting: "That's what they were there for, to clean up other doctors' messes." That was an understatement.

On Sunday I got my schedule for the next week, and I noticed that the next Friday I had the same meeting with my team of doctors. But what I didn't understand was at the bottom of the Friday square, it said moving day. What was that?

I was sleeping better because I was so exhausted from everything, but I noticed that lady was in the class about vocal chord dysfunction and some other classes, and that's when we started greeting each other. But I was really into working and learning, and at the time, that's all I wanted to do. Everything didn't always go perfectly, but what in life does? Friday came around and at our meeting there were different people.

Everyone who had been working with me was there, but the only one that bothered me was the woman psychologist, and was she going to discuss things that we had talked about. I should have known better than that. How stupid.

The one thing that I didn't know about was they were moving me to a hotel a little ways from the hospital. I needed to see on my own what I learned and start cutting the umbilical cord. The hotel and the hospital were affiliated, and if something went wrong, they would call the hospital and send a PA and a nurse, and if they thought they needed to get you back to the hospital, they would oversee that. Otherwise, they had several buses that went back and forth all day in order to get to the hospital for the classes and all the other things.

At first I was so scared that all I wanted to do was lock myself in and come out when Monday rolled around. I then remembered my cousin lived around there, and I called him. He came over Sunday, and we went for a long ride and then ended up at his house for supper. I didn't want to leave, but he walked me back to my room. The day was so fantastic, and I was glad I remembered he lived there. Greg was what I needed at the time, and I thank God he was there

Greg, like a gentleman, walked me back to the room. I went in and I thought that I saw that lady that I had seen in the bar, so I went to investigate. She was there, and I asked if I could sit with her, and shortly after that, we had become friends. We had a few classes, and we both ended up with vocal cord dysfunction. We both had a lot of anger from the news.

What is Vocal Cord Dysfunction?

Vocal cord dysfunction, known as VCD, is hidden but common and often misdiagnosed. It is an unsuspected condition of throat closure and/or choking sensation that can strike any age. In the ER, VCD is usually misdiagnosed as being difficult (refractory or brittle) asthma (severe, life-threatening allergic reaction) or hysteria.

An article by Carol Sidofsky explained it the best way I could ever think of. VCD is like breathing and straining through a straw; some can't get air in or out at all. Panic and fear of dying from the feeling that one isn't getting in enough air often causes repeated ER visits or hospitalizations.

The throat closure actually occurs inside the voice box (larynx), behind the Adam's apple, when the vocal cords go into a closing-up spasm.

Some symptoms are severe asthma, severe allergic reactions, collapsed lung, pulmonary embolism, actual choking, something obstructing or narrowing parts of the airway, and spasms of the diaphragm muscle.

A laryngoscopy directly looks at your vocal cord. I told you that it was neat to see my vocal cord.

The only thing is I used to love to sing and I can't now. Speech therapy helps!

No medications are used, but on me the damage already had been done.

The following week, I worked so hard and the psychologist and I would kill two birds with one stone by walking and talking at the same time.

This next part of the story, I'm not real proud of myself. I had thought of suicide twice. Once was shortly after that severe attack and another time when I came home from the withdrawal and the muscular pain was so bad that I didn't think that I could handle another day like that. My psychologist wasn't surprised or shocked. But she asked where I stood at the time, which was better. Then I told her that I thought I was coming here to die. I also told her about the Friday I told Dean I would walk off the plane and into his arms. She thought that was great, but she hoped I didn't set my goal too high; then I showed her what I found in my suitcase when I opened it in my room. It was a picture of Angie with a note that said, "Don't forget me, Mom." I think we both had a tear come out of our eyes.

Back at the hotel in the evening, several of us got together; some would have a drink and some didn't.

One evening, I had decided to go back to the room, and I noticed that the elevator was already open, and I still was watching how I was walking with the cane. All of a sudden, a voice said, "Miss, could you possibly back out and wait in the lounge?" There were three firemen with all their fire equipment on going to a fire on the tenth floor. Then a person from the hotel said that we could go back to the lounge for drinks on the house. I still felt pretty dumb, but everyone got a good chuckle out of what had happened.

The last night, my friend and I walked over to Applebees for dinner, and we sat there a long time, and I was wishing she lived closer than Pennsylvania;

I think we would have been very good friends. We were both excited to think that in twenty-four hours each of us would be home.

The next morning was another consulting time about everything that I would need for swim therapy, a psychologist that my doctors could get me into, and lastly about my adrenal gland. But you can't imagine how much better I felt; they told me that I was through the worst, but the drugs would be in my system for a while, and I had to be careful. I then said my thank yous, but how do you tell someone thank you for saving your life? In 1997, I would come across that question again.

We caught the shuttle to the airport, but before we left, we enjoyed throwing all our medicines away.

I went out on eight medications and came home on three—prednisone, blood pressure medication, and lots of calcium. My suitcase was lighter, and I brought back my breathing machine.

When we arrived at the airport, we said our goodbyes, and off we went, different ways and back to our lives at home. I remember forgetting to say thank you for making time go faster and that I enjoyed her company. She was a hoot.

When time came to board, I went on early with my cane and all. I knew the man standing in the door where the pilots were, and I looked at him and he stood up and said that I looked so much better, and he asked if I was going home and I said yes. This was the pilot that helped me get settled that early morning when I thought life wasn't for me anymore. I told him that I would be walking off the plane.

When the seatbelt sign came back on and we were getting ready to land in Wichita, he sent a message back to me asking if I wanted a wheelchair just in case. I said no. Everybody was in such a hurry to get off the plane, and I didn't take any chances. I got to the door to start down the hallway when the pilot was waiting and asked if he could escort me off to my family. I wanted to cry but accepted his arm. I then saw Dean and Angie looking out the airport windows. We got out the door, and he said I was on my way. I went right in Dean's arms, and a hug from Angie didn't hurt either. I told Dean I loved him and Angie thanks for the picture and note. Then I cried. I knew that the last two years were over, but what I didn't know what was just starting.

SEWING WITH MOM

Mom was always interested in helping Dad out with the bills. Her parents had given her some money for Christmas, and she bought a Singer sewing machine in a nice cabinet. This went into the den by the north window opposite the piano and Dad's desk. This is also where she did her ironing. Then she bought a book on learning to sew and taught herself to sew. She took a few classes and went to work. She had that knack for being able to read a book and then she could just do it. She was a perfectionist.

She started making dresses for me and then with the leftover material would make my Barbie doll dresses. Sometimes we girls would look like triplets. She would sew every free minute she had; if there was hand sewing, such as hems, buttons, etc., she would sit in the evenings when we watched television and work on things. She believed in the following the pattern and ironing the seams down when she finished sewing the seam. If she didn't like it, she would rip the seam out and do it over. Oh, to have one day back when we were trying something on and she was busy pinning. All she would say was, "Don't move or you will get stuck." We got stuck, so we believed her.

I remember one Christmas when I got a Barbie doll case for all the clothes that had been made. The case was blue with many Barbie dolls posing on the front. Opening it up, there was a place to lay Barbie and next to her were two places to hang her dresses and there were three boxes for drawers under the hanging clothes. They got me a lot more shoes to match the dresses. I never had too many original dresses since she made everything that I wanted or watched me in the store looking at outfits. Everywhere I went, my Barbie case went with me. Eventually I collected Ken and Barbie's kid sister, Skipper, and Barbie's friend Midge. Mom and Dad called me a packrat. But I had to pick everything up when I was done or it was time to eat. I didn't like to do that.

Another year, when my grandparents were coming for a visit, usually two weeks in the summer, Mom thought that she could make us all outfits and have our picture taken together. First, she wanted to find the right material. Then she saw some Hawaiian design in green and white and thought that would work. She made dresses for me, Grandma, and her. Then made shirts for all the men to wear with their white pants and white shoes. Barbie wasn't left out either, and Mom went to work. All her spare time was working on all that material, and finally the day came when the open area where the guests coats went was filled up with shirts and dresses in that Hawaiian, green and white material, and was she proud; we all were.

The day came for the picture, and the ladies looked really nice because Grandma bought us each white beads to finish off the outfits. The men, on the other hand, were having trouble buttoning their shirts. All of a sudden, Mom discovered she had put the buttons on the wrong side, but once they were buttoned it didn't show, and she couldn't redo that mistake because she made the buttonholes on the machine.

She had made three men's shirts, each in different sizes, and they looked handsome. Our grandparents took us out to dinner after the picture had been taken; we didn't go out to eat much during this time and that was a real treat.

Mom was left-handed, and I learned a lot of things left-handed, like ironing and dealing cards. Hand sewing was a little hard, but then Grandma Ethel taught me a lot about hand sewing, and I changed over to using my right hand, and when Dad saw me peel potatoes with my left hand, he just couldn't believe it, but that's the way I was taught. Now, I can really peel potatoes; if one hand gets tired, the other hand takes over.

I think one of the last projects of sewing was when Mom made a suit for my nephew, who was three, and a long dress for my niece, who was four. They were my ring bearer and flower girl in my wedding. They were so cute. Then Mom seemed not to sew very much because of the way the RA had effected her hands. That was the end of a great hobby. It was unfortunate how her hands got so knotted up.

When they moved into town, she didn't want to get rid of her sewing machine, so they put it down the basement, and when the girls and I went there for a visit, I would make several outfits for my girls. Angie loved to play with Barbies, but it made me nervous making all the little seams, and Angie played with my Barbies with the blue suitcase, just like I had many years ago.

The Sewing Machine

After Dad had his cancer, they couldn't take care of the yard, and the house was too big. They moved into a condo with two bedrooms. They had to auction lots of their valuables away, but Mom still couldn't part with her sewing machine. Instead, she got the idea of using it as a place to put her makeup on. She wasn't sewing much any more, due to her hands. She couldn't bear to sell it. She had it all organized and we always knew where she was around 8:30am.

In the last house they lived in, her makeup was still sitting on her old sewing machine until the day she died. Dad decided that he wanted an apartment, so there was no more room for the sewing machine and the original cabinet. I couldn't let it go, so I asked if I could have her mirror and everything that went with it. Dad was pleased that I wanted it. So that old Singer sewing machine, in the same cabinet, sits in our bedroom where the makeup mirror sits with her makeup mirror and my makeup.

Girl Talk

When we would sew together, we used to call our time girl talk, and usually the men would just roll their eyes and leave the room. Mom read everything she could get her hands on, especially *Good Housekeeping* magazine. One time, she read an article on how to straighten your hair, and my hair was naturally curly and I hated it. So Mom and I decided to try it. We ironed my hair; it worked and would stay straight until the next washing. Then when I washed it, she always had a pony can of beer to put on after rinsing it. I would let it sit on my hair for thirty minutes and rinse it out, or we used lemon juice or eggs to make it shine. She used mayonnaise to help put moisture back in her hair because her medicine would dry her hair out, and these were things we had around the house.

When I was little, every Saturday afternoon, she would wash my hair in the bathtub, and when she used to rinse it, she would put my head under the faucet and I thought that she was going to drown me, so when dad came in for coffee, he would hold my finger and stayed with us until my hair was washed.

We really did some strange things together. Another time, she found out that I was smoking at college, and one afternoon when I was home from school, she asked me to have a cigarette with her. She and Dad still smoked one with a high ball while watching the news. This about killed me, and she thought that I would quit but that didn't work until a couple of years later when I was first pregnant with Jennifer. I threw up for five months. When anyone smoked around me, I would have to run for the bathroom, and I had quit by the time I had Jennifer. But any smell would have that effect on me. We had our girl talk all though the years, and in a following chapter, you will hear about the best girl talk we ever had.

THOSE TEENAGE YEARS

There was a time when I didn't want to leave my mother's side. Gary was the type of kid that enjoyed going exploring and wandering in somebody else's house and flipping on the TV. Mom was upset because Dad was due home. But they found him because he left the door open. They always said, "Gary wasn't worried; he knew where he was at." I, on the other hand, wouldn't let go of Mom. I went through more purse handles from holding on so tight. But as the years passed, it wasn't always that way.

I wonder now why in the world I did not like her very well. Don't get me wrong; I always loved her. But I was a real brat.

I can't remember when I started dating, but I was always really embarrassed by introducing her to my boyfriends.

My parents never minded boys coming around; in fact, I had several boy-girl parties when I was in seventh and eighth grade. Once, Dad met everyone at

Charla Johnson's house with the tractor and hayrack with lots of hay and took us out to the farm for a barbecue and dance in the yard. Another time, Dad, Mom, and I cleaned out the barn and had a barn dance. Two weeks later, they had a dance because it looked like fun. There was a cement floor and once cleaned, we would sprinkle cornmeal, and it made the floor really nice for dancing.

Yes, there were times when Mom didn't seem to know anything and I did. We went that route a lot and poor Dad was always in the middle of us.

Mom was always a perfectionist, especially when it came to cleaning the house on Saturday mornings. My job was to vacuum and dust the upstairs and dust the whole downstairs. I tried everything to just get by, but she always caught me. Dusting is still my least favorite job, but she would even do a white-glove test but with no white glove. She always found dust under the dining room table or on the rungs of the chairs. I couldn't stand her for that. Can you actually believe that she said she was preparing me for my house someday or for my children? When she sat me down to tell me the facts of life, I would almost run off from her. (I was faster, anyway), so when I was home from school with the flu, she would get the books out and sit by the couch, and I thought that I was sick already, give me a break. I was going to fool her; I wouldn't have a period, and just for that, I'd stay with them the rest of my life and make life miserable, just like she was doing to me. But Mother Nature took over, and

I felt that everyone was ganging up on me, especially when I started in math class wearing a white skirt.

The worst time is when I would get a "downslip" or a report card that I wouldn't brag about. She always thought that she was so smart, that I could never please her. Boy, what planet did I come from? I had a problem with school, and she couldn't accept it, but if I was in school when my girls were, they would have found a learning problem, and they'd think it was hereditary. Everybody thought that I just wasn't too smart and that ugly word was used: *dumb.* Well, I wasn't dumb; we got over that, but when the girls had it, I worried all over again, but it was handled so differently, and Mom even felt bad, but nobody knew.

Thinking back now, maybe if she should have kept the communication lines open more, but then we wouldn't have been the friends we were in later years. But she could always get the best of you!

Between my junior and senior year, I started dating this one guy, named Duane. My mother was so excited. She thought I had really caught a good one. But that didn't stop me from still looking around. Debby always kept the game book at the city baseball games. Finally, I started meeting her there. Now, I looked a whole lot different then, and I remember watching *The Sonny and Cher Show* and what made Cher's shoulder shine when she had a halter shirt on. Well, baby oil worked for me. I always saw this one guy, but Debby said that I could never get him; he was out of my league. Debby and I were sitting and talking to someone in the concession stand when this one guy came up and got a pop. I looked at him just as he looked at me, and even though it was summer, I had chills that ran all the way down me. Now, explain that.

Anyway, the hot dog I was dating was okay, and I stayed with him. Dad really didn't have much to say about him. Several weeks in to dating, we were supposed to go out after I attended a wedding with my parents. But his brother called me and said Duane wasn't going to make it. So that night I picked Debby up and went riding around. I was given a good shock; there was Duane, riding around with another girl. That was the first time I had a broken heart. I was really upset. But we were riding around, and I was licking my wounds. We kept going by this one house, and finally these guys yelled at us to come over. We did, and funny as it might be, it was the guy who gave me the chills, and his name was Dean.

Class: Friendship 101 - Debby

It seemed that Debby was with me when important things happened, but I suppose that is what a friend is all about.

Debby has been mentioned several times in this book, and to this day, our friendship is still there. It's different now, but Debby taught me a lot of things. I don't quite remember when we started hanging around together, but I know it was in high school. Mom always thought she was so funny and used to laugh at the way we ate salads. Our specialty was a lettuce salad with cheese and bologna and, of course, dressing.

We did a lot of strange things together, like when I took her out in the country and taught her how to drive a truck and shift gears. I got down and worked the clutch, brake, and the gas. She got the rhythm down between the clutch and the gas; it was funny that we didn't burn the clutch out. While we are on driving, I would be driving, and all of a sudden, she would be sitting on the window outside of the truck and waving at everyone. We always had a good time together, especially when we pulled in for gas at the Farmers Union and gave this one guy fifty cents in pennies and he would stand there and count them, so we could look longer and talk with him. That bought almost two gallons of gas. We took turns doing that.

I don't think you would call us daring, but we can honestly say that we never got drunk; we had more fun without getting drunk.

We always went everywhere and did everything together. One summer, we enjoyed working on old furniture and learning how to antique the wood. We liked that green color of antiquing and did everything we could possibly do.

But she was there the night that Dean finally called. After that night, we talked to Dean and his friend Dave. I thought that I wouldn't hear from him again. The following day was a Monday, and I was working with Mom while her assistant was on vacation for her daughter's wedding. I had to go back to the doctor's office. I was getting tonsillitis every couple of weeks, and the doctor decided to take them out on Tuesday. The tonsillectomy didn't go well, and I ended up staying longer in the hospital. The day I came home, Mom and Dad had a meeting to attend. Debby came to stay with me. I don't remember if my throat was back to normal, and I had just gotten out of the hospital that day.

I hadn't heard anything from Dean, and Debby and I were discussing what she heard Wednesday night at the game. The phone rang, so Debby answered the phone. "Sundberg residence, Swenson speaking." Her eyes got so big, and I asked who it was. It was Dean, wondering if I could go out with him on Sunday. I asked Debby if she thought that Mom and Dad would let me go out. We were so excited, and this is what I mean; she was there from the start. She would be my maid of honor; I was her bridesmaid; she is godmother to Angie, and both her daughters and mine were in the same grades. She was in the ICU at Wichita with Jennifer; we went over to see her when her husband died. Our friendship has changed a lot through the years, but I think that's because we grew up, but there are a lot of things that we did that I won't put down in black and white.

Changing of the Times

When I started dating Dean, I was young, but Dean and the previous guy were the same age, but Mom always thought that Dean was a little fast for me. I think Dad liked Dean; at least he never said anything. But somehow I fell hard for Dean, and then he decided to sit out a semester of college and work for the state highway.

My parents were very stern about seeing him. I got to see him two nights during the school, and we didn't go anywhere but watched TV on my parents' couch, but that didn't seem to matter as long as we saw each other. On the weekends, we went out on Saturday night and spent most of Sunday together. Of course, I had to be in at a certain time on Saturday night, and we were always at the house, but we would actually sit out on the porch or the patio and talk until my mom started yelling out the window or turning off and on the yard light. I dreaded January; I knew he was going back to college, and I figured that back on campus, he would see the mistake in dating me and go back to his normal routine. He bought me a beautiful watch for Christmas, and I bought the first gift I had ever given any man. I really loved this guy, and if he had asked, I'd have married him in a second.

January 1974 came and I couldn't stop it. The night before Dean left, I told him that if he got back and found out that he didn't want to be with me, at least be honest and tell me. Our age difference was five, almost six, years. He really got upset with me and asked if I didn't what to see him anymore. Then he told me his plans of coming home every weekend. I couldn't believe it; he also said that he was in love, but I already knew from the third date.

Mom told me not to put my hopes on this working until she had talked to one of his married friends at a coffee party after a high school basketball game. She was told that Dean had really changed in the last six months and that he was serious about me. Mom couldn't believe what she was hearing. Then on Friday evenings, he would drive in at 5:00 p.m. on the dot. She knew then that this was for real.

I thought that when my graduation rolled around that Dean would give me an engagement ring, and I was kind of hoping too. But he gave me a beautiful necklace and had popped the question. We held off telling anyone until March 1975 when my parents announced our engagement in the paper that we were getting married September 6, 1975. When Dean graduated with a BS degree in geology, we had written and sent letters out for jobs. Dow Chemical replied back, and he had an interview and got the job but started in July, two months before we were married. With the help of Steve, his brother, we went to Enid and found our first apartment. It wasn't far from work, and I liked it until the neighbors drove me nuts, and I really wasn't used to town living.

When Dean had left for Enid, Mom and I were busy shopping and preparing for the wedding. She and I would shop all day on Saturdays, picking out everything from my wedding dress to what I was going to wear on my honeymoon. That was kind of embarrassing.

While Dean was working in Enid, Dad, Mom, and I worked on the invitations, which had to be mailed out on my birthday, August 16, 1975. Then I made sure that the best man and groomsmen and Dad had been fitted for their tuxes. One night, my parents and I made and molded all the mints for the wedding. Dad enjoyed this part, and we found out they were harder to make than we thought, but we figured it out and they turned out fantastic. The butter mints were my favorite.

Dean and I had already gone to the classes with Pastor Mo and had our blood tests done at the doctor's office, two weeks before the wedding. I took our birth certificates and blood test results to the McPherson County Court House to get the license. That wasn't the problem; the problem was picking it up. When I went to pick it up before Dean got home, I asked for the marriage license for Dean Elmquist and Wendy Sundberg, I never looked at his birth certificate, and it wasn't there. So I did a slow panic, they punched in the date of marriage and found a Charles Elmquist instead. He had always been known as Dean, and he didn't like Charles, but I didn't know that. I paid, took the paperwork, and got out of there because of the stares I was getting; the best one was from the head clerk. I bet he was wondering if I even knew who I was marrying.

Our wedding was beautiful, except Dean had a hangover from the night before. Kraig, my nephew, did really great at the rehearsal, but when the little guy saw all the people in the church, he said, "No, way" and wanted his daddy. LaShae, my four year old niece, on the other hand made it to the altar but started eating her flowers during the service.

I then put Dean's ring on the wrong hand and the wrong finger; he waited until the wedding was over and his finger was turning blue, just like our colors, but we survived. I would have done really well if I hadn't seen my aunt; then the waterfall turned on.

Dean took me to Enid the next Tuesday because he had to be back at work the next day. The following week, he left on a Monday and didn't come home until Thursday night. I had no car; I walked to the Safeway around the corner and was ready to have our marriage annulled. Boy, did I get broken in as an oil field wife and hated it. There was a friend, wife, and their new baby that lived not to far from the apartment. Dean knew him real well and he was in my brother's class in high school. I babysat for them, and they took me shopping, and I learned how to macramé. After the first Christmas party, I got to know some of the wives, and they had some of the same complaints.

One wife told me that they stopped over to see if Dean needed any help cleaning the apartment before I got there. When she walked into the kitchen and saw the mess, she just asked Dean over to dinner and told him nicely to clean up the kitchen at least. He threw out all the empty chicken boxes and bags from other meals and kind of cleaned the refrigerator out, but cleaning was not his thing.

I was pregnant by our first anniversary, but before that, I kept getting sick and couldn't shake the flu. I was throwing up at the sight of food and just felt horrible. Finally, I went to see our doctor, and he said I didn't have the flu, but I was pregnant. I then said, "How did that happen?" He looked at me and made the comment under his breath that I was one that was going to keep him up all night. I didn't understand until I went into labor.

There had been a lot of improvement in the relationship between my mom and I during my pregnancy. I was scared about having the baby, but I had a lot of time to think about being a mother. Mom and Dad came down around my seventh month, and we spent the weekend getting the baby's nursery ready. While Dad and Dean painted, the ladies worked on curtains. I bought a sheet with Raggedy Ann and Andy because I thought that would fit for a boy or girl. Mom helped make the cutest curtains, and we had a great day. Being a mother is not the easiest job in the world, but back then I also needed a friend. That Sunday morning, Mom and I went walking, and I felt like she wanted to tell me something. I could tell that whatever it was, it hurt because her blue eyes were bluer. Dean's mother had told my mom that she couldn't figure out why Mom was coming down after the baby was born and not her since she had taken care of a newborn before and Mom hadn't. I couldn't believe what I was hearing, and I felt bad for Mom. Mom said that I could change my mind, and I refused to discuss anything more on the subject. But I asked Lenore if this was said, and she admitted it to me. I think that started the problems with Lenore for the rest of her years.

Two months later, after Dean had stitches in his hand, my parents came down again hoping that I would have the baby sometime that weekend. Everyone had told Mom to walk and that would get labor going. So we walked all over the neighborhood, and when Dean came home from work, we walked over to the park, which was less than a block away. Dad and

Dean were looking at something, and Mom was with them while I sat on a bench. For late March, it had been a beautiful day, and I decided to go down the slide, and I didn't have a problem going up the ladder. Then I pushed off and got over the first hump and came to an abrupt halt. I was stuck. How was I going to get out of this mess?

Mom turned around and saw me sitting on top of the second hump, wondering how I could stay there, until I told her that I was stuck. Her eyes got huge, and I had seen that look on her before. I told her that I thought that I would be having the baby soon; then you could see the panic. I told her that my hips must have been getting ready for labor. She soon understood but didn't help getting me off the slide. Finally, she walked up from the bottom and somehow got me unstuck; she then sat down and went down backward, and I stopped her from landing on the ground. By this time, the men were running toward us, and then I got yelled at.

The next day, Mom and Dad had to go back and were disappointed that nothing had happened. Dean was called out on an overnight job. I went to sleep early, but around 7:00 a.m. woke up, and my water was starting to break. I called the doctor and went in for a checkup, and guess what?

DEAN

Dean had grown up in Lindsborg, just as I had. By writing this book, I couldn't believe how many things that we had in common. Our fathers went to Lindsborg High School and were in the same graduating class. So we had the same reunion pictures until Don passed away. Our mothers worked in the same office, and I guess this is where Mom had heard how wild Dean was, from his mother at coffee time.

Dean worked for my dad, baling hay on the farm.

I had known who Dean was and remembered him talking to a girl at the swimming pool. I thought he was good looking then.

I sat between his uncle and aunt when I sang in the church choir and never knew they were relatives until my grandma told me. She and Vi had been friends though several clubs at church.

Dean and his brother, Steve, grew up in a home that wasn't always happy. The boys were little when they moved in with their mother's parents, and their grandparents weren't very well and very hard to manage.

Don was a good father. He had fought at the Battle of the Bulge, and family members said he was the same when he came home. He started drinking but wasn't ever mean. He would work through the week and kept a bottle by his chair on the weekends and then was ready to go to work on Monday. His drinking progressed, and he would go on binges, and Ken and Vi (his sister and brother-in-law) would have to find him and bring him home.

After a while, Dean's grandma passed away, and his grandpa was put in a home. Things got better, and Lenore became pregnant and was hoping for a little girl. Their daughter was stillborn, and Lenore couldn't handle it, and she was put in a hospital in Topeka, Kansas. Don continued to drink, and eventually Vi and Kenny took over raising the boys. They had a lot of good memories by living with them. They lived on a farm, and their aunt and uncle were always playing a joke on each other, and the laughter was great for the boys at that time.

Lenore got better and got to come home, and things went well for a while until a day in early 1963 when Lenore and Don got together with friends in Salina, and Don and John decided to go fishing. The call came in that one of the men had a heart attack while fishing and were at the hospital. Neither of the women knew if it was John or Don until they walked into the ER and saw John waiting for them. Don had died on the way to the hospital. Dean was eleven, and Steve was twelve.

Their lives changed from there on, but both boys graduated from college and became good fathers.

After Lenore died, we were going through some paperwork, and we found papers from Don's time in the military. We found an envelope to Lenore from the Office of the President, and it was recognition of his service, and I'm sure that every veteran gets one, but it was the signature of the president that caught us off guard: John F. Kennedy in June 1963, and in a few short months, he was assassinated.

Dean is a good father and enjoys being a grandfather. But Dean always wanted me home with the girls and didn't want me to work until they were almost in junior high. It was important to him that the girls always knew I was at home waiting for them, and this wasn't always an easy job. I basically was their only parent because he was gone so much.

But this man that I was lucky to marry has been so good to me and for me. Our friendship has been very loving, and we have had thirty-four years of life together.

JENNIFER MARIE

Jennifer was born March 29, 1977. I was going to be twenty-one on my birthday the following August. I enjoyed having someone to look after, and I wasn't by myself anymore. I always felt like she was going to be a girl, even though Dean was hoping for a boy.

She started walking at nine months and was climbing out of her bed to where we let her sleep in the guest bed on the floor.

She was a climber. She got hurt on some things, such as the dresser in our room, and it tipped over on her. She was always kind of accident prone, just like I was.

As you see, she has the name Marie too. Well, we had to carry the name on. I always thought that it worked real well with Jennifer.

When Jennifer was young, she always had an ear infection; I had them too. Finally, we decided to put tubes in her ears. In the late seventies, it was more of a surgery. We checked in the day before and stayed the next night after surgery. Believe me; it was a long two days, and it seemed to work, but I had to wash her hair at the sink so no water would go in her ears. I never let her play in the tub either, which always made her mad. But I knew she could hear. I ran the vacuum shortly after we came home from the hospital, and she screamed because she had never heard that sound before. Reading to her was so much better because she sat and listened, like all her books were brand-new.

We were both lonely for Dean, and now, looking back, I think this is why she never slept well until she was two years old. I never let her sleep with me unless she was sick or had a fever.

Dean was home on my twenty-first birthday and decided to take his girls out for dinner. But it turned out not to be a great birthday. Dean had called me from work and told me to go to the bank and draw money out for my birthday dinner. He had gotten reservations at a nice restaurant. As I carried Jennifer into the bank, it seemed like everyone was acting strange, and I couldn't figure out what the problem was. Dean had beat me home and was waiting for me to pull in the driveway; then I heard the news. Elvis had died. That evening, we didn't need the reservations because there was nobody there. Dean felt bad, but it wasn't anybody's fault. But when my birthday comes around, I know there will always be Elvis movies on.

Jennifer loved going to Grandma and Grandpa's farm. Grandpa would take her on the riding lawnmower, and she called my dad "wa haw." I think from the time she was a baby, that's what it sounded like because of her ears. But she took a real shining to my dad. She had good taste in men. From day one, they had something special.

My parents came the day we got out of the hospital. I was so shocked to hear that Dad had gone shopping on his own and bought her a purple lacy dress with matching purple shoes. Dad always left the shopping to Mom. She looked like a little Easter egg, and I kept the dress and shoes.

After Jennifer's first set of tubes came out, the ear infections didn't go away. One afternoon, her temperature went up so high and fast that she had a seizure. This scared me, so as soon as the infection was gone, we tried the tubes again. Finally, we made headway and kept the infections away for more than a year. The next set was done with removing the adenoids. This finally worked, and she became so much stronger and healthier. We thought that we had finally conquered Jennifer's ear problem. Life went pretty smoothly for a year until the summer between kindergarten and first grade. It started out when she hit her head and had a very serious concussion. After that, she seemed to get very accident prone. Our family doctor said that when I would call and it was about Jennifer; he would want to see her because whatever happened, she was hurt. Dean and I noticed a change in her but could never put it together until about a month before Christmas; this was the accident that started the nightmare.

The PTO always put on a Santa Store where there were nice gifts the kids could buy with their money. The student body always looked forward to when they could go shopping, but first they got to see what was in the store and view all the items. That afternoon was Blue Birds for Jennifer's class. I had my helper with me, and Angie always enjoyed being along. Then my name came over the intercom and said to go to the gym ASAP. I grabbed Angie and ran to the gym. Jennifer's class was leaving, and the I saw people with Jennifer as she was lying on the floor below the stage. The principal and gym teacher said that Jennifer had fallen off the stage, but she went straight off, and her body landed flat, and she didn't block her fall. She looked like she didn't know what had happened. She was very confused and scared.

I took her right to our doctor; she had cracked her cheekbone, broken her arm, and had numerous bumps and bruises. Dean got to the office while they were putting her cast on, and the doctor explained that we needed to start investigating and running tests. He thought that over the Christmas holiday would be the perfect time.

We went to Lindsborg for Christmas, and everyone was there. Dinner was over, and the kids were getting antsy about opening presents, except for Jennifer. Gary noticed that Jennifer was very quiet and sitting by the fireplace watching the fire. He walked over to her and sat by her. She was very warm, and he scooted her back. He noticed that she didn't even attempt to move, and it was like her body was stiff. He called me over, and we both started to talk to her softly until she came around, and afterward she was exhausted to the point of opening presents wasn't real fun.

I had that gut feeling that something was really

wrong. At the hospital, a CT scan, EEG, and lots of blood work were done. Then the test results were slow coming back because of New Year's. But Dean and I had an appointment with the doctor the following Monday in the afternoon, except I was called to come to school. The principal had taken over the class because the first grade teacher had gotten the flu. He had noticed Jennifer having some type of staring problem and that they were lasting longer each time. I rushed Jennifer back to the doctor's office, and they let me come in the back way. Once in the office, she had a major seizure, and my first thought was to try to yell at her, which didn't work. They had her in an examining room and finally thought it was better to ask me to step out. That was the last time I ever left the room. I was sitting in the doctor's office, and Dean came in for our appointment and was shocked to find out that Jennifer was there having seizures.

It seemed like time stood still, and finally the nurse said we could see her. She looked horrible, and I started to cry. The nurse told me to stop or I would have to go back to the office. If she had came out of it and I was standing there crying, she would have thought that something was really wrong and it would scare her. Well, you try to stand and look at your child and her not knowing who you were and not cry.

As she rested, we went back to the office with the doctor, and he started reading her test results. He cleared his throat and announced that Jennifer's EEG was abnormal, and I didn't understand what he was saying; then epilepsy came out of his mouth. I just shuddered.

She was admitted to the hospital and given medication. She continued having the seizures until finally we got her on the right dose, which took two weeks. Mom and Dad were there, and I remember that Mom and I were sitting by her bed, and Mom said, "God doesn't give you anymore than you can handle."

I honestly didn't believe that at the time. We went to several specialists, and they didn't want her to ride her bike, swing on the swing set, basically do nothing at all because she could get hurt. Finally, we had to have her schooled at home. I kept thinking this was all wrong, and I had done some studying on the subject. I learned about the whole field of epilepsy, and I felt that we were missing something. It seemed that Jennifer got more seizures at home, and she was very depressed for her age.

Finally, with the help of my dad, we found a pediatric neurologist in Wichita. We had an appointment within weeks. I didn't like going over anybody's head, but I wanted answers. After one appointment, we knew he was what we needed. Jennifer fell in love with him. He said to let her grow up and not to hold her back, that this was causing her more stress and aggravated the seizures. Kids get hurt and that was a part of growing up. She told him that her medicine tasted nasty after she took it. He said it had a aftertaste and showed her what he did. He showed her a case of LifeSavers, all cherry, and he said to take one after her medication; he also didn't quite agree with the medicine she was on. Every time we left his office, we always felt better about everything.

Jennifer eventually ended back in Wichita and was admitted to the pediatric ICU for many days. I was glad we were close to the family and friends; it helped time go faster. When my dad and I went in to see her, he'd hug her so tight that it kicked off all the machines that she was hooked up to. He was also there the day they took her IVs out and while holding her, she accidentally pottied on him, but he didn't seem to mind because she was alive. We ended up on the pediatric floor, and she and I roomed there for two weeks. She had a small incision on her head, and they were watching her closely.

Dean, Angie, and Lenore went back to Enid when Jennifer had stabled out. Dean needed to work, and Angie needed to be back home and back in her routine. I knew they were both being taken care of, and Dean called us every night.

Jennifer attended school at the hospital, so she didn't miss a lot of schooling. Finally, she was down to one medication, and she was more responsive to everything around her. The doctor came in one night and wanted to take her off the last medication to see what would happen because her EEGs were showing that her brain waves were almost normal. I asked him what had happened. He told me that the brain takes care of itself, and if there is a part of the brain that's damaged, another part will take over. We don't use half of our brain, and sometimes there is no reason to what the brain can do. Medications seem to cause more problems. What caused the trouble, we will never know.

For some reason, the last medicine gave her the most problems, and she ended back in ICU so they could watch her. That evening, I couldn't go back to our room to rest, and then I wondered if I did the wrong thing. There were a lot of what ifs. Finally, at the start of the second day, she was so much better, and we went back to her room. She started right back to school and was eating, drinking, and everything was working right with no medication in her system. We were absolutely shocked at the difference; she was the old Jennifer that we lost three years ago. Our family doctor didn't see how this was going to work, but the day had been set for going home, and we were ready. Dean decided to take a week off, and when they came to get us, he just couldn't believe what he saw. My parents were there with Lenore, and when we were ready, her doctor came in and reminded me that Jennifer was going back to a different world. She wasn't sick anymore, and the faster we got her back to school, the better she would do.

We were so scared taking her home. We needed her to know not being sick; she couldn't wrap us around her finger anymore. This was not the easiest time for the both of us, but as time went on, we settled back into life. As she finished up grade school, she was tested many times on how to handle life and handled it, and then we stopped wondering about the what ifs. This wasn't easy for us. But with the help of her doctor and all the follow-up appointments, together we handled it. Everybody was so excited when it was the first anniversary and then the second and the third and finally the day her doctor decided it was time: her last appointment. We knew he would always be there if needed, and he was excited; there had been another girl about Jennifer's age that had the same problem and went home on no drugs. It doesn't happen very often. But I was glad that it happened to Jennifer.

Today, this time in our lives is simply a memory, and Jennifer has had no seizures, but once in awhile she has a migraine. She knows the onset and starts on over-the-counter medication and two warm cokes. This opens all the blood vessels, and the migraine medication seems to go to effect faster.

The Teenage Years

Jennifer had a real hard time when we moved back to Lindsborg when she was going to be a freshman. I kept telling her that she would enjoy being in a small school and having friends. Well, one thing I learned during this time was you never can go back. Just because Angie had an easy time with the move, why would Jennifer? And at this time in her life, I made many mistakes.

After she turned sixteen, she got a job at the Swedish Country Inn. This really helped her self-confidence, and soon after, she bought her own car. The banker really expressed how he was going out on a limb by loaning her the money; he read her the riot act. I thought what right did he have, and it was her parents that would be watching over her. I was pretty angry and thought about going to where we banked instead, but Jennifer stuck right in there and paid the car off three months early. She asked me to go with her when she paid the last payment, and she wanted the banker to accept the check.

We went in the bank and waited. Finally, he wasn't busy, and we entered his office. Jennifer explained that she wanted to make the last payment on her car early. He was at a loss for words. She handled herself very well and kind of put the man in his place. Self-confidence. No problem. It seems funny now because she has a very high position in a bank and loves her job.

As for boys, she learned the hard way to be very picky about who she went out with, and I always thought that she would end up with an age difference in the man she would pick.

By Jennifer's junior year, she seemed to overcome her learning disability on her own, and I'm still not sure how she did that. The only thing that bothers me is that Jennifer had so many events put on her, such as my illness and how she took care of Dean and Angie while I was gone, that she seemed to get cheated out of her teenager years. She always acted older than she was.

Jennifer found her way through life. She basically stopped eating, and I never noticed it until one day in the bathroom. I can't believe how clothes cover up so much. I wanted her to go to the doctor, and she told me she wasn't sick. I let her have some room, and I didn't want to eliminate any connection of communication with her, and this was difficult.

I finally got a call from Jennifer at school, and she was very upset. I checked her out, and we had an appointment with the doctor, but I let her go in by herself. I felt like this was a cry for help, and we got her that help from a very smart lady who was a psychologist. She wanted to see Jennifer in her own setting and came to the house; they also had sessions by going and having something to drink. No medication, and all of a sudden, Jennifer started back on food but at her pace. This took many months, and there was a lot more to the story, but Sally found Jennifer for us.

Jennifer started letting friends back in her life and started getting out more and just being a teenager. She and a girlfriend started going to a dance club in Salina and learned how to have fun. This is where her life changed, and she met the man she would spend her life with. Meet Howard.

Jennifer Meets Howard

Howard was stationed at Fort Riley in Junction City. When Jennifer told us that she had met a soldier and he was coming to see her, Dean and I looked at each other. Our thought was that the soldiers from Fort Riley were out for something, and boy, were we off. But he pulled up with a friend and instantly became one of the family. We could see how smitten he was with Jennifer, and this was the first time in a year she had given a guy a chance. They started dating, and he finally bought a car from a soldier on base and started coming every Friday. Eventually, we found out that he had already served in Desert Storm and Panama.

Being from Louisiana, I wanted to make holidays special for him. For Thanksgiving, we had our usual, so Howard could meet my parents. At the dinner table, my dad asked Howard to pass the butter, and he kept saying "Yes, sir," and finally Dad said he didn't have to say that, and Howard disagreed. My dad had a higher rank, and Howard said that was a form of honor. Boy, did that stop everyone from eating, but Dad felt so honored. I thanked Howard afterward for what he said as we were washing dishes, and he said he didn't need to be thanked; that is just what he was taught—respect.

A couple weeks later, the four of us went to the Christmas tree farm for a fresh tree. Jennifer and I picked out the tree, and the men told us that it was man's work to cut it down. Back at home, they carried it in and put it in the stand—man's work again. Then Jennifer, Angie, and I started putting the lights on when the tree and the stand, filled with cold water, fell over on us. Jennifer finally crawled out from under the tree and said, "Yep, that's man's work," and it sounded so funny. We had a mess to clean up, but it was done with the Christmas spirit.

Jennifer finished up her senior year. Howard was on maneuvers. My dad was in the hospital, recovering from cancer and a stroke. We were remodeling the bathroom and kitchen, which was a mess, and she was really stressed by all the things going on. Dean and I had planned to have a reception for her at my parents' house. She was happy by then because Howard was waiting for her as she came out the door following the graduation, and he was what she needed.

Two of Jennifer's teachers came, and they were her favorite teachers. Mr. D was the chemistry and math teacher. He was my teacher too, which really makes this story because he said every time he would call on Jennifer it was like I was there, and he would call her Wendy. Debby's daughter was sitting by Jennifer, and they always laughed because every one wanted to know the deal with Wendy. The girls, of course, both knew and would laugh. She said it was easier to answer instead of having him embarrassed. More or less, she let him off the hook, but just like me, she learned a lot from him and also Angie had him, and he was in the top two of her list.

Then came another story. Her next teacher told us about something that had happened the last day for seniors. He was walking down the hallway and rounded the corner and was met with a soaker water gun. He said that Jennifer was one of the dream students, never caused a problem, always had done her work and handed it in on time, and was very quiet. It never bothered her to be called on in class. He said it made teaching very easy. But Jennifer was on the other end of the water gun. He was soaked and shocked; he just couldn't believe it was her. I asked if he had handed in the grades yet.

Jennifer attended Bethany College for one semester, and Howard had proposed to her. They were planning a summer wedding when he got notice that he was going to school in South Carolina and then he'd be transferred. So the wedding was pushed up to February, and it was such a nice wedding that people still comment on it now. Since it was the day after Valentine's Day, we made heart-shaped cookies and bought chocolate kisses for each table. Everyone enjoyed sitting around and watching the kids open their gifts. It was a wonderful evening.

Howard left four days later, and Jennifer, Angie, and I had a great time together. We didn't know where they were going, and I wanted the days to have time with my girls. We sent Jennifer to Howard so she could see him graduate, and then once back in Kansas, Howard found out they were going to Houston, Texas. They lived in an apartment until they bought a beautiful home. Those two had a lot of fun. They went to all kinds of different events, and when we came, they went out of their way to show us a good time. We went to see the Titanic exhibition and saw Cher in concert. We enjoyed shopping in Galveston and at Keyma, walking the boardwalk, and just having a good time. I hated that she was so far away, but I was glad she got to see things she had never seen before.

Six years later, our grandchild was on the way, and they allowed me to be with them when we welcomed Landon to their family.

After the birth, they thought that Houston was not the place to bring a child up and decided to move back to Lindsborg where their children could grow up with the luxury of grandparents, great-grandparents, and an aunt. They moved in with us. Jennifer was able to transfer with her job, and Howard found a job since he left the army after ten years of service. I babysat for them, and things worked out pretty well.

We decided to find a house and buy it together. It was very difficult to find the right house, and our poor realtor, we ran him all over the area until he found this house for us. He sold our house, and the kids sold their house in Houston. We weren't sure about moving out of Lindsborg, and I worried about leaving Angie and our parents. But we downsized and moved in the house on July 5, 2004. Our first major problem was an ice storm that hit, and we had no electricity for a week and ended up at my parents' condo for five days. It was like camping. Then Jennifer was pregnant with Lucas.

Things have worked out nicely. Dean has retired and helps me with the boys. Everybody goes his or her own way, and we have our time and they have their family time. We see Angie and Dirk, and they visit with us. We do enjoy staying with them at their home and also when they need someone to babysit their dogs, Dexter and Pup Pup. So, all's well that ends well.

The Diaper Story

Let me tell you that from the time my girls were born to now with our grandsons, absolutely nothing has changed in the poop department. Newborns still have that nasty runny poop that can shoot clear across the room if you're not careful, especially when they are being nursed. I think that this is one of God's jokes on women. He gave us a way to feed our babies, but he knew that it had to come out the other end, and that's when he thinks it's funny and probably when it comes out both ends at the same time. Well, that is just hysterical to him. By this, let me tell you what happened.

Shortly after Lucas was born and Jennifer was nursing, we all tried to sit down to dinner, which was a tough thing to do. We were trying to resume our lives, pre-Lucas.

We smelled something that wasn't dinner, and it was time to change his diaper. So Howard said to go on and eat and he would take care of his son. While eating, we heard a yell for help, and I volunteered my services, which was my first mistake.

I still remember running through the kitchen and into the boys' room. First, I asked Howard what was needed, and then I stepped up next to Howard at the changing table. The second mistake was being at the wrong place at the wrong time.

Howard had attended to the cleaning up of the dirty work and was ready to put another diaper on Lucas. All of a sudden, it was like he exploded and shot poop out, like he was aiming at someone. It went everywhere on us; it was horrible. I jumped back and fell over Landon's Weeble Town and all the Weebles. I fell face first and hit my head on the edge of the bed. By this time, Dean and Jennifer came in to see what all the commotion was about. I was lying in the middle of the Weeble park with about thirty Weebles driving their cars or playing on the swing set or just lying there. I felt like the man in *Gulliver's Travels.* Jennifer helped me up and was still laughing hysterically. Dean was in the background giggling, and Howard asking what I was doing.

They helped me out to a chair in the living room, and my toe was bleeding and everything ached. I had baby poop all over me, and there was even an area on the carpet that showed where I had landed. I had Weebles everywhere! I slept in the recliner and didn't even bother to clean up. The next morning, I took a hot shower, and I had little bruises all over from the Weebles. I asked Jennifer how much damage I had done, and she, still laughing, said none. All the town of Weebleville survived. So you know now that those toys do not break.

A couple days later, the stiffness was gone, but I woke up with the biggest—I might add prettiest—black eye you have ever seen. The next day was our anniversary, the thirtieth, me with my black eye. We went to Target, and the cashier asked how I got my shiner. I told her the story, and she laughed so hard that someone had to take her place. I had all these little red marks that turned into black and blue marks, a really great black eye, and everyone was looking at me and still laughing. We discuss that time and Jennifer starts laughing all over again. Funny!

STACEY LYNN

Stacey Lynn is our second daughter and will always be the middle child. She never got to come home from the hospital. We will never forget her.

I didn't get to hold her while she was alive, but I heard her cry. She was in Dean's and my life for such a short time, but she has always remained in our hearts. No one should ever have to bury a child.

My first three months, I felt great and wasn't even sick a day, like with Jennifer, which was a real plus. We were so excited at this time because we were in the process of buying our first house, and in my fourth month we moved in. While packing, I was standing to where Dean saw a side view of me, and he made a comment about not showing. I had all the normal signs of being pregnant and my OB was watching me closely. He thought it was a normal pregnancy. But a little voice kept telling me something was wrong.

When we moved into the house and things got settled down, we wanted to do some remodeling to the house. But we put that on the back burner. We went ahead and put the crib up and kind of organized things then. We met our neighbors, Mr. and Mrs. Ernie Chambers, a wonderful retired couple. Ernie had been an electrician. Every evening they would sit out on their porch, and I would usually bring Jennifer over to play in their yard. It sure made time go faster while Dean was gone.

By the time I almost was in my sixth month, I started having problems and was admitted to the hospital on complete bed rest. Dean took time off to take care of Jennifer. My parents came down on the following Friday night and talked with the doctor before they saw me. I was excited; I had gone twenty-four hours with out spotting. When Mom and Dad entered the room, Mom started crying. I thought that maybe her RA was acting up and probably wasn't the time for a long car ride.

I went home and straight to bed, and this was where I was going to stay until the birth. Mom and Dad were taking Jennifer home with them, and I hated the thought of not hearing her laugh or her playing. Dean told me it was for the best, and he had hired a girl to come in every day to take care of the house. I guess I had nothing to worry about. Mr. and Mrs. Chambers were going to look in on me too.

Mom had been very emotional her stay in Enid, but I had seen her like this before. But when I walked in the door, Dad, Dean, and George P. (from work) were putting a new floor in the bathroom and carpeting it. Dean was trying to get the bathroom fixed up for me. I could see it from the bedroom and commented on it all the time. I was watching them work from the bed when all of a sudden all three men were tripping over each other trying to get through the door. I was puzzled, and then they started laughing. Our Norwegian elkhound, Huck, had come up under the house and stuck his nose through a hole, and the men thought it was a rat.

The next day, my parents left with Jennifer. They left early so they could get Jennifer home and settled. I cried myself to sleep; she had been my whole life. I felt empty. Dean had a few tears but left me alone. It was so quiet, very lonely.

By Monday everything was back to normal. Dean was on a job, and the girl was supposed to start on Tuesday. But Ernie came over and visited for a while. Dean came home, and I told him that I wasn't feeling very good. I had some strange cramping. The doctor had recommended that I could have a glass of wine, and I went off to sleep. The next morning, I felt bad, but the girl was over for four hours, and I looked forward to that. By the evening, I called a friend and discussed with her, and she thought I should check in with the hospital. I called and they wanted to see me. She drove me and said that she noticed the way I was walking and that something was wrong, and the nurse thought the same thing. My water broke, and labor was on. I never thought that she wouldn't be okay, and Deloris called and got Dean right in. He came up, but I told him to go home and rest. They would call if I needed him, and then I tried to get some sleep. At 2:45 a.m. I was ready, and I had no medication. Miss Stacey was born at 3:15 a.m. Dean missed the birth. I knew something was wrong; too many people were around her and that made me afraid to look. She had come, sack and all. Dean saw her when she was cleaned up. No facial hair, but she had the Elmquist nose, weighing in at one pound, one and a half ounces, and eleven inches long. Dean held her; her chances weren't good. She had a IV and oxygen, but she was really having a hard time.

We decided to help her but if she started the dying process to let her go. No suffering. Dean stayed with her until the last fifteen minutes of her life. He came in my room and told me and then sat in the corner and cried for a bit. I wanted to hold him so bad, but he didn't need me at the time, so we waited. She had been baptized and given the lasts rites and died on July 11, 1979, at 6:00 a.m. I got to finally hold her for a while after they wrapped her in a blanket, and the doctor took care of everything else. But we had a little time with her, and I remember looking at her and thinking she looked like one of my dolls in the past. She was cold, and I remember cuddling with her, but she was still cold.

The funeral home came, and it was time to say good-bye. I hated how he put her in a basket to carry her to his car. I asked if he could just carry her out of the room so I didn't have to see her go in a basket. They did what I asked. The doctor decided it was time to give me something to sleep or sedate me. Dean called Mom and Dad; they couldn't talk but would call back a few hours later after I had some rest, and Dean went home. Ernie was standing on his porch when Dean pulled in the driveway and said he would go to the funeral home with him. Dean didn't know what to do. Deloris' husband was with Dean, and all three men went down and made the plans. Deloris was in the recliner next to the bed, and as I woke up, she was there to cry with me.

The plans were made. We were picking her up on Friday and taking her home to Lindsborg for burial in the Smoky Hill Cemetery by Coronado Heights. My grandpa was the president of the cemetery at the time, which helped with the paperwork. He and Dad marked off a plot and dug her gave. The ground was very dry and hard to dig, but they thought that was the least they could do, and anyway Grandpa wanted her in the family plot. Dean and Bill went out and bought Stacey a doll dress and a beautiful blanket for her, and then they went shopping for carpeting for the rest of the house and brought me the samples to look at. Everyone went home around 4:00 p.m., and fifteen minutes later, there was a knock at the door and Ernie came in. He said his wife was too upset to come and see me, but he had seen Dean come home and thought I was alone then. He said he was so sorry and all the plans and paperwork were done. I thanked him for everything.

That evening, I called and called Dean, but nobody answered. Finally, he showed up and told me the house was too quiet. He took down the crib and put it away. Then he went to see the new James Bond movie *Moonraker*. The first movie he took me to was *Live and*

Let Die with the new James Bond, actor Roger Moore. He got away from the phone and watched the movie by himself. He climbed in bed and went to sleep until the nurse woke him up.

The next day, the sun came up, and Dad had called. He told me that they got permission to put Stacey's casket on a table in front of the altar for the night. We both had a hard time talking to each other, and all I wanted was to hold Jennifer. Dean came in with a dozen red roses, and the doctor was right behind him. We talked, and he wanted us to know that at this time it could make or break our marriage, and if that started to happen, we should call him. He would make an appointment with someone to talk to. He asked about the plans, and Dean told him. He said that he was sorry they couldn't do more. But I knew it was out of their hands, and she was in a much better place. We have never wavered on our decision to let her go.

I couldn't understand about Dean bringing the roses to the hospital, but when it was time to leave, I was sitting in the wheelchair, and as they opened the door to my room, he put them in my lap. I had something in my arms to carry out of the hospital. I couldn't believe he thought of that.

At home, we packed and got ready for the next day's trip home. The Carters and Mr. Chambers went with us to the funeral home. They wanted me to see the casket before the next day. Until I saw the casket, it had been just another day, but this had our daughter in it. It was a shock.

July the thirteenth was on a Friday; we hadn't thought about the date. We were getting ready and had the TV going, and on some morning show John Denver was singing a song that broke both our hearts. We gathered everything and went to pick Stacey up. There had been flowers delivered to the funeral home, and Dowell had sent a beautiful arrangement to my parents for the church. They carried the little white casket with pink bows to show that the head was there. They carefully put it on the seat in the back. We collected all the paperwork to bring a body over the state line to Kansas. Their secretary came out with a box of Kleenex, which we didn't have but could use. Off we went, and both of us were very emotional. The tears dried up by the time we reached the interstate. Dean and I didn't say two words to each other until we got stopped by a highway patrolman.

This was not good; Dean had been speeding, and we were caught. The patrolman walked up to the car with his sunglasses on and asked for Dean's license and insurance. Dean said he was sorry and to just give him the ticket. I think that's when the officer noticed our puffy eyes and the flowers in the backseat. He pushed his sunglasses down on his nose and saw the casket. He was shocked and his voice wavered; he asked if we had the proper papers, and Dean handed him the envelope. He handed the papers back to Dean and then thought what his next words were going to be. He ripped up the ticket and told Dean to watch his speed and that we really didn't need a ticket at this time and told us to go. That was the longest three-and-a-half-hour drive.

Arriving at the church, Dean carried Stacey into the church and set her on the table with a beautiful lace cloth. We sat there for a while, thinking over the day and deciding that this was all we could do for her. We left but didn't know that Dad was in town waiting for us to leave, and then he went in and sat with her for a while. He then knew I needed Jennifer and went to the babysitter's and picked her up.

We stopped to see Mom at the office before leaving for the farm. It was very emotional, but she told me that the night at the hospital when she saw me, she knew what was ahead of me; she knew I would lose the baby. She felt so guilty feeling that way, and when it actually happened, she really felt bad. But she felt like she had been prepared in order to help me. Dad and Jennifer pulled in the driveway shortly after we had, and I was never so glad to see her, but sitting on the patio, all she cared about was playing with her toys.

The next morning, we were up early because the funeral was at 9:00 a.m. at the church. The arrangement of flowers had been delivered from Dean's company with a check from passing the hat around. Gary and his family were in Illinois visiting family, and Dad didn't call him until the night before the service.

Everyone who was invited to the service was there, family only. We took a couple of minutes outside to get ourselves together when the minister came out. He had confirmed me, married us, baptized Jennifer, and now was performing the service for our second daughter. It was all a little too much to handle. Knowing everyone was in their seats, Pastor Mo escorted Dean and me to our seats, not too far from Stacey. His service was around thirty minutes, and then everyone followed our car to the cemetery. Mom held the casket on her lap, and Pastor Mo sat beside her. It was a beautiful, cool morning; we stood around the grave that Dad and Grandpa prepared. Dean and I put two roses on the casket. At the end, Mom asked everyone over for coffee and goodies. Dean, Dad, Grandpa, and Dean's brother stayed and buried our little girl. I often think about that; Stacey's father, grandpa, great-grandpa, and her uncle laid her to rest. Grandpa said at the coffee that he should have never been beaten to the grave by his great-grandchild, but in these changing times, no man will ever hurt her; she was in God's arms. Pastor Mo announced that her baptism was on the book in the church and that we could always look up the date, July 11, 1979—born, baptized, and died on that day. She will always be remembered, though she was only on this earth a short time.

When everyone left, Dad and Dean went to town and picked Jennifer up at the sitter's and brought her back to the farm. It was time to go on. About six months later, I felt like I went through it all over again when her stone was finished and I saw it printed on the stone. But I still have her birth certificate with her footprints on the back. One foot had an arch, and your thumb would cover the one footprint with space on each side. Dean brought me the pink bows off her casket, and they are in her memory book. I visit her, and Mom is now buried right beside her.

We stayed for a week, but Dean needed to get back to work, as if nothing had happened. Jennifer and I were back on our own, and I was afraid that she would leave me too, so I kept her very close. I realized that having any more children wasn't going to happen, and maybe Dean should find somebody else. Everything I tried to do, he stuck in there with me. Finally, he got me interested in remodeling the house together. This is what we needed, and we finally got through the after effects, together.

ANGELA JEAN

I was scared about getting pregnant again, but I found out the reasoning to what happened with Stacey, and it would have happened again. There were new things out to stop it from happening. New medications that slow the cramping and pain down. It wasn't going to be easy, but Dean and I thought about having one more child.

I never had a problem getting pregnant, and the first three months, I rested more, and I had a purse string put in the opening of the uterus and pulled closed so there was no way I would have this baby come out until it was time. I did have more appointments, and labor started and stopped several times. At those times I thought that it was over, and I was going to lose this baby. I couldn't travel or have company, extra work, or excitement. Every day was another day I marked off my calendar.

I was due around the first week of July, but in May, my grandma was admitted to the hospital. Dean and I had talked to her on the Sunday before she died. She told me not to come or take any chances. She seemed to know that I was going to have this baby, and she was excited for us. Dean teased her about sounding good, and she needed to go home. She did want to go home, but Monday night, she passed away. Mom called the next morning because she wanted me to sleep. This was my first grandparent that died, and I missed her dearly. I was pretty low for a couple of days.

Dad wasn't doing well after everyone went home. Grandpa did real well, and now he had to talk because Grandma always did the talking, and he was quiet. I should have been home helping out, but I couldn't leave the house.

In 1981, the ultrasound was just starting to be used, and knowing the date of birth wasn't as good as it is today. We missed the date they gave me, but a couple of days after that, my labor started, and the OB decided to take the stitches out. They thought that I would have the baby right away. When that didn't happen, we went to our second plan. I would go home, and the labor would start. The doctors didn't think I would be home long. The third plan was an appointment every week, and after two and a half weeks, I was still pregnant. Dean thought that the baby had taken permanent residency, and I actually was very miserable. I couldn't get cool, and I was past the middle of July. Finally, my blood pressure was getting high, and they did a stress test, which came out fine. A week later, the morning of the twenty-third, was B-day. They started my labor, but nothing was happening, and Dean had gotten in from the job and decided to eat because at 7:00 p.m. the doctors decided to go a head with a C-section. Dean and I were watching the news, and my back was sore from lying around all day. All of a sudden, I told Dean I felt something, and he looked and called the nurses. He saw the head of our baby. Did we cause a commotion then. Angela was born at 6:45 p.m. They cut her nails before they cut her cord for fear that she would scratch her face. We kept hearing a strange noise, and the nurse said she was sucking on her thumb loudly. We had a thumb-sucker.

Dean called home and really caught everyone off guard and thought I must have had the fastest C-section of all time. Good thing we were at the hospital, and then I remembered that it would have been my grandparents' sixty-second anniversary. This was the way it was supposed to happen for my grandma.

We soon had our family home, and Dean thought that everything would get back to normal. What he didn't know was that it was just starting. Angie really looked like Dean; the doctor even told him that he couldn't even deny this baby because of her looks.

The only argument we had was her name for the birth certificate. I wanted to name her Angela Dean, and Dean said he wouldn't pick us up at the hospital if I wrote that down. He picked out Angela since I thought of Jennifer's name. So I decided to name her Angela Jean.

Dean took ten days off. Dad had been in and out of the hospital, but they came down shortly after we had gotten home. Dad wasn't good, and his skin was a gray. He didn't even want to hold Angie. Six weeks later, the girls and I went home for a week. Dad was in the Salina Hospital, and they didn't know what was wrong. He was transferred to Wichita, and they found a degenerative nerve problem and started fighting it with medicine. He was out of the hospital and home in two weeks and back to his normal self. Angie's first Christmas was good, but we still missed Grandma. I always felt guilty about not being there, but look what we got out of the deal, and I did what she wanted me to do.

Angie was a whole different baby than Jennifer. Jennifer never started sleeping through the night until she was two and a half years old. Angie loved her bed; she took two naps a day until she went to kindergarten, and she was ready for bed at 8:00 p.m. She was slower to walk and wanted to stay in her crib instead of a big girl's bed. I never knew if she would take her clothes off and run around nude until Jennifer would bring her inside. Jennifer called her "a nudey baby." She loved it when her daddy was home and sat with him in the rocking chair until she dozed off, and he tucked her into bed. She never once tried to climb out of her bed and loved to play with Barbie dolls at a young age. She would chew on their feet and eventually one foot would be missing.

I bought new cape cod curtains for our room because we moved into a larger brick home before Angie was one, and I thought that they looked nice from the street until she cut holes and made Barbie dresses. She said she loved the color blue and thought it would look good on Barbie. Dean took her out to work a few times to do his paperwork, and they called her "Teenie Deanie" because she looked so much like her father.

Angie was always very social and had lots of friends all through high school. She was excited about moving to Lindsborg and fitted in nicely. She only complained of two things: she missed the skating rink in Enid, and we couldn't take our dog, Nelson, with us, and she hasn't forgiven me for giving him away yet. I think that Gary described her perfectly; if we all looked at the world the way Angie did, there would not be any wars. She always looked at life and she said it the way it was and she still does that. She cracks me up at times, and it seems as if everyone is waiting to see what she says next. For instance, she started calling Jennifer "Fo Fo" and when we were in Walmart buying shoes, she let one right by Jennifer and then said, "Excuse me. I fluffed." So when we met up with Dean, she told him that she fluffed, and he replied, "That's nice." I told him later, and he about came unglued. You never knew what was next.

When Jennifer was dating Howard, this was the first time Angie had a "brother" around every weekend. She was going out on a date, who is still a friend of hers, and Howard met him at the door. Howard was an army soldier and stood over six feet. He told Angie's date that he would hurt him if he tried anything with her. It was a joke, but he scared the young man. Jennifer made him apologize; I don't think he ever came back.

When Jennifer and Howard got married, Jennifer and Angie bought her maid of honor dress together. They did a good job; it was a slinky red dress that showed every line. Angie showed up at the church, and Jennifer told her to take her underwear off and just wear hose. They yelled back and forth at each other until Angie stomped into the bathroom and yelled that Jennifer was making her take her underwear off, and of course being in a bathroom, it echoed. She then said she was going to walk down the aisle and stop to tell everybody that Jennifer wouldn't let her wear her underwear. It sure made Jennifer nervous for a while, but everything turned out fine.

Angie really missed Jennifer when they moved to Houston, and one spring break we flew her to Jennifer for the week. They went shopping for prom dresses since Angie had a date. Jennifer wanted something different for her, and Angie came home with a beautiful dress that she got to wear many times. They had a good time together.

When Angie graduated and went to college, she stayed in town but lived in the dorm. She was undecided on her major and thought about teaching and took her teaching block. Angie had the talent of drawing anything. She went through a time where she didn't know what she wanted and had some trouble, but she decided to go into art and loved making pottery. She worked very hard, and without the teacher she had, she wouldn't have made it. We never saw her too much, and my parents said that she was estranged, which they meant they never got to see her.

She and her friends were in a sorority, and her friends were great and we never worried very much because she was very particular whom she hung around with and whom she dated. There had been a few guys, but she knew what she wanted and wouldn't settle for anything less. This is where the girls were the same, which kind of surprised me.

She also had the same learning difficulty that Jennifer had, maybe a little worse, but we had help for her in high school until the day her test scores were in and her counselor from the state of Kansas told her that she would never make it through college and that she should go to a trade school. The way he said it, well, I got mad because for being a counselor, he never was in touch with her after they first met. She graduated in 2005, and it took five years, but she had changed her major midstream. At her graduation party, she invited her teacher from high school and wanted to invite the counselor too since he lived in Lindsborg, and she wanted to rub salt in the wounds, but we told her she had nothing to prove.

We went on vacation to Disney World. She moved back in the house from the dorm. She told us that she had been seeing a student that was going to college, and he came from Hillsboro, Kansas. He was a music major. The curtains were closed, and as he rode up on his bike, I knew who he was from working at the college. His name was Dirk, and I didn't think he had a chance. Dean and I made a bet on how long he would last. Two weeks later, we went to Orlando, but she had bought a calling card and called him a lot.

When school started back up in the fall, they were together a lot. He came over with her a lot, and we really thought that this was a nice young man and were embarrassed about the bet that Dean and I had made. After 9–11 happened, we decided to go to Houston and spend Christmas at Howard and Jennifer's place, and they hadn't met Dirk yet.

We usually spent the night and made it a two-day drive because of my back. We stopped and asked if they wanted their own room, and they said that they would stay with us. Then we heard the funniest thing, Dirk has a beautiful voice, and he always sang in the shower but he danced too. We laughed, and Angie said that he never sings the same song twice. The next day, Dirk was introduced to the rest of the family, and he fit in so well. We had a wonderful holiday. We always made Dirk take a shower in the downstairs bathroom so we could hear him sing.

Then after spring break came the time you don't ever want to think of. It was a Sunday afternoon, and Dean had something going on at the campus. Angie and her girlfriend came over, and as we were talking, Angie said that her and Dirk were going to be living together. They had rented a condo with several of their friends. She was twenty-one, and I couldn't really say much, and Dirk was getting ready to graduate. When Dean came home, I told him about Angie's plans and agreed since she was of legal age she could do it, but he didn't have to like it. Dirk proposed on September 6, 2004, our anniversary.

Things worked out, and they had a beautiful wedding in July of 2005. When Mom started her decline and was in the hospital, Angie started stopping by and watched TV with them and just got to know them again. They would always start looking for her shortly after she was done with work. She would spend a couple hours with them and decided to stay with the same job since it was in town. In October, they rented a house in Salina because Dirk had a job there, but Angie refused to leave her job in Lindsborg for the reason of checking in with her grandparents.

They both have good jobs and are very happy and quite comical together since Dirk is six feet three inches and Angie is five feet three inches, always a foot apart. They have bought their home and are happy living with their two dogs, Dexter and Pup Pup. We enjoy spending a weekend with them once in awhile.

Last October, all eight of us traveled to Disney World in Orlando for a week. We had such a great time, and it was fun to watch how the boys took in all the parks. We finally got to see the parks through the eyes of the children.

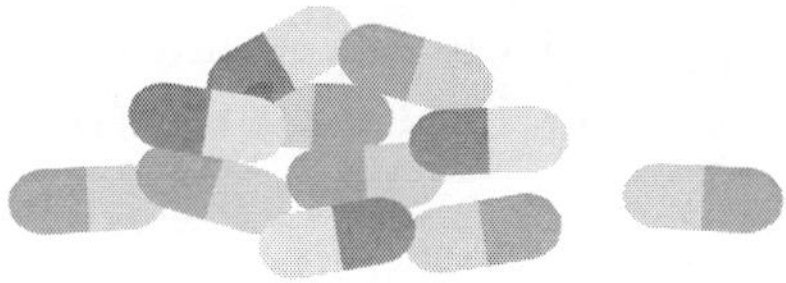

LIFE IN ENID, OKLAHOMA

Dean took a job with Dowell, a subsidiary of Dow Chemical. He stayed with this company for sixteen years. When the oil field started to slow down, the name changed several times, and at the end, it was DS. Believe me, this was not an easy life for him or us.

They paid well and gave excellent benefits, and we always knew that there was somebody on the phones in case we needed our husbands in. We were called the "oil field widows," and the oil field was like a woman; she always tried to get the men away from their wives, and lots of marriages didn't make it. All the hours they were gone, it wasn't worth it.

The company supplied their uniforms with their name on the front and the company logo on their backs. We used all the washing and drying time for a deduction on income tax. The uniforms were made of Nomax for safety and were fire retardant. Dean used to say that the uniforms were warm in the summer and cold in the winter. The first couple washings of the uniforms smelled the whole house up, and they were hard to get clean because of the Nomax. I spent a lot of money trying to find a cleaner that could go in with the soap. The best thing I found was by accident. Jennifer had left her coke on the washer, and it fell in with his uniforms. After I dried them, they looked brand-new, so from then on I used coke, and it worked like a charm. Have you ever thought of your stomach? But I couldn't complain because the company supplied them, and Dean was safe. He never brought his uniforms in the house, and we had a place for him to dress and undress in the garage. He was so dirty when he came home. He couldn't wear a ring or a watch because he could pull his finger or arm off.

One morning, the girls were getting ready for school, and Dean was on his days off. I went out to start his work shirts, and I had a laundry hamper for his dirty clothes. As I went to grab a shirt and felt something soft and furry, and I thought that one of the girls' stuffed animals got thrown in with his clothes. Then I looked down and saw two beady eyes looking up at me. I immediately walked to our bedroom where Dean was and told him about the eyes. He laughed at me! When he went to take a look, he pushed the hamper over, and there was a possum that had taken up residency in Dean's uniforms. Dean shot back in the house and told me to call someone. I called animal control, and they came right away. They got a noose around her neck, and she automatically grabbed the pole they had. She was either very pregnant or had them tucked under her tail, but I wasn't going to look.

They took her out in the country and found a place for her. So we understood why she was a bit nasty.

Our brick home was in a fairly new housing development and was one street over to a wheat field. I enjoyed living and raising the girls in this area, and we were also on the boundary for school districts. The Enid Board of Education decided to have a school bus that took the kids in the neighborhood to school and back.

Now, I think back about how nice it would have been to have cell phones. That would have helped talking more with my husband, and the girls could have talked to Dean too. That might have even helped some of the marriages. Even having a laptop would have been great.

Before we had the girls, there were a few things that happened, and the first one was when Dean had been out over twenty-four hours and had gotten around three to four hours sleep only to be called back out. What Dean didn't know was that the day before, I was cleaning the bedroom and decided to change the bedroom furniture around. When the phone rang for his wake-up call and he went to answer the phone, he went into the closet instead of the hallway. First, I answered the phone, and then I helped Dean find his way out of the closet. All our clothes were strung all over off the hangers, and some of the hangers were wrapped with the clothes. He had tripped all over the shoes, and I'm not for sure, but I think he fell down several times. Once he was awake, he was not happy with me. I thought that I needed to clean the closet anyway, and from then on when he called and said he was on the way home, I would tell him that I changed the furniture around. He told me later that he felt like he had walked into the twilight zone.

Another time, and the best one, was with the dispatcher who was doing the wake-up calls. When he called to wake Dean up, I told him that Dean had already left for the shop. The dispatcher was mystified and told me that it was the first time he called. I told him that Dean wasn't there, but all of a sudden I heard Dean's voice, and as I looked over, there he was, looking at me very strangely. I told the dispatcher that he was there and handed him the phone. I had just had a dream that Dean had already left for a job. When Dean got to work, the dispatcher wasn't sure what had happened. He said that I had him convinced that Dean was already on his way to the shop. All the guys thought it was so funny, but the dispatcher still wasn't clear on what had happened. I just kept them guessing.

After moving from the apartment to our first home, I felt like we were living in a cabin. It was really neat and had a big yard that was mostly a big hill. All the cabinets were built in, and we didn't need any dressers. We moved in one load, kitchen and bathroom stuff, a beanbag chair, and a rocking chair. For eating on, we had a card table and chairs, which worked great. We bought a bedroom suite from some people at Dowell. When we went home, there were some things from each parent that we brought back, and it turned out pretty cool. I bought several cement blocks and antiqued some boards and made a stereo shelf, and all of a sudden the house started looking like a real home. The next item on the list was a baby crib.

Someone at work said that his mother-in-law wanted to get rid of the crib she used for her grandchildren, so I called her, and we went to see it. It had been new but with very little use. She was really fair on the price, and the mattress came with it. I had looked at cribs, and they were as expensive then as they are now. We had to take it apart to get it home, and Dean went right to work on it. Cribs are hard to put together and to make sure that everything worked on it. When it was done, I helped him push it into the bedroom, and it was too big to get through the door. So Dean took it apart and redid it in the bedroom. We felt pretty silly. We remembered that every time we put the crib together again.

The hill in the backyard was hard to mow during the summer, but in the winter, we had a lot of fun. We would invite friends and their families over for a sledding party. We usually just had snacks and hot chocolate, and we had no sleds. Cardboard was great. When it snowed, everything kind of shut down. They couldn't get to locations, and when it snowed, it really snowed.

Everywhere we lived, we always were lucky and had nice neighbors. A nurse lived at the first house. She was working on learning to paint. I found a picture that she had trashed, and I really liked it. I had it matted and framed in what looked like barn wood, which went with the theme of the picture. It is still hanging on my wall, and when I look at it, I think of her.

We bought our first house in 1979. It needed work and remodeling, and it was going to be slow because I was pregnant with Stacy. This was the project that we took on together after Stacy died.

Dean and I learned a lot and eventually had fun working on the house.

Our biggest project was going to be the kitchen. We needed new cabinets, countertops, sinks, flooring, and whatever else I could think of. We had gotten together with four couples one evening, and how the subject came up, I don't remember. Basically, the men bet the women that we couldn't get the cabinets down before they went on their three days off. The bet was if the ladies won, the men were going to dress up and take us out for dinner. I don't remember what the bet was if the men won, but it didn't matter.

The day before the men were off, we got together, and one of the women knew all about carpentry because her father was a carpenter, so she was the foreman. The bottom shelving pulled out pretty easily. The kids were real good for us; we had just bought a VHS, and I rented a bunch of movies for them. We put a baby gate across the door of the kitchen. We took care to turn the water off and plumbing for the new sink. Luckily, we had all the new stuff in the garage, and we did our measuring, and everything went so well until we were taking the top cabinets down and pulled the wall with it. We all looked at each other, and there were the studs of where the wall used to be. So two of us went to Sutherland's Lumberyard and bought what we needed to fix the wall. We also bought electric wiring for an idea we had. We fed the kids and sat and thought about our next move. We wrote everything down and went back to work. Before the new wall went up, we wired for two new outlets and a light above the sink. I went next door and got Ernie to come over and take a look at our work. He thought that we had done a nice job, and the wall was up. We cleaned, mopped, and even carried the cabinets in and waited for the ladies on the porch who were having a beer, and the kids were sleeping on the floor. The kitchen came out great, and the men were astonished by what we accomplished. We won the bet. We eventually sold this house, but the biggest problem was that the closet was huge but shared by two bedrooms. Jennifer had gotten in a habit about not knocking on the door to our bedroom, so Dean put a lock on the door. It worked great until she started coming through the closet and asked what we were doing and if she could play. No comment needed.

Our next house was our brick home, and we lived there the longest. It had three bedrooms, one and three-quarter bathrooms, a nice size master bedroom with a walk-in closet, and no one shared a closet. It also had a two-car garage and a fenced-in yard. The girls remember that when they were old enough, I would give them each some money and they would walk to the Kwik Shop a couple blocks from home. The only problem was a bare spot in the front yard by the driveway. Nothing would grow, and I thought that maybe the builder dumped something there so the grass wouldn't grow. Little did we know there was a story about this place.

Jennifer loved shadow boxes that hung in her room; she collected little stuff, which ended up as her hobby. Angie had them too, but she didn't keep them like Jennifer did. But Angie always loved Jennifer's boxes but could only look, not touch. She would quietly go into Jennifer's room, and once in awhile, she would accidentally break something. She was scared and sneaky at the same time. She would either bury these items in the spot out in the yard, or depending on how big they were, bury them in the sand box. She always just played by herself and used her imagination, and now one of her nephews can sit and play by himself. He doesn't always want to play with his brother, just like Angie was.

I bought a paddle at a craft show, and I hung it in the kitchen. Whoever painted it did a great job on it because it was called "a fanny whacker." I didn't use it much on the girls, but they knew when the fanny whacker came off the wall and was in the chair in the living room, they had pushed me to far. They usually disappeared into their bedroom or straightened up and flew right. It disappeared, and I looked everywhere for it. Finally, I decided that it would show up somewhere in time, but it never did. Angie admitted to me a few years ago that she had broken it and buried it in the sand pile. What kids will do.

The girls had their share of pets, but the best one was Nelson, the Bassett hound. He was really cute and cuddly, but he was very stubborn. Nelson and Dean didn't get along real well. We always had a burp rag lying around because when he would shake his head, you almost had to duck for cover because slobber would come flying out, and it was kind of disgusting. Bassett hounds are known for this problem, but we didn't know this, and we got one that had the problem badly. The girls and I started to call him "slobber doggy."

When the oil field went bad, Dean was one of the last eight to get let go. A year later, we sold our house and rented a nice house over by where our first apartment was. There was a fenced-in yard, and there had been a place behind the garage where there had been a garden.

I started digging the garden up, and our neighbor came out and we got to know each other. He thought that Nelson was one of the funniest dogs he'd ever seen. Perk and Laverne were our last neighbors in Enid. They were a lovely couple. Perk had worked out at the airport, and Laverne sold material downtown at a fabric store where I used to buy material. One afternoon, they invited me over for coffee, and as I walked into their front parlor, there were pictures up on the fireplace, and I couldn't place the woman in the picture. When you can't place someone, it really bothers you. I enjoyed being with this couple, and they knew when we were outside because Perk would be outside or sit on the porch with us.

We had our lawnmower a long time, and we thought that it was on its last legs, and at this time, it wasn't what we wanted to spend our money on. Perk saw that Dean and I were working on it, and he said that he could fix it. He worked on it in his garage, and a couple days later, he brought it back over, and it worked like it was new. We wanted to pay him, but he never took any money from us. But when I baked cookies, I always brought them some.

Then as my garden started growing, he started helping with it, and for such a little plot, we would give at least half of the neighborhood fresh vegetables. Perk and Laverne, lived in the neighborhood, most of their married lives. They never had any children. But we sure kept them busy until it was time to move to Lindsborg, and they hated when the moving truck packed up our things.

But first, back to the pictures on the fireplace. I finally asked Perk when Dean and I were over for coffee. Perk told us that it was his cousin who used to fly airplanes and even had come to Enid to visit him. Her name was Amelia Earhart. This is how he got interested in getting his pilot's license. Perk's last name was Earhart. He hated when the anniversary of when she went missing came around. He always felt that something went wrong, and the sea got them. The pictures were wonderful, and the one that Perk had was of her standing by her plane with her navigator; it gave her life as we had never seen. He never thought that she was still alive and living somewhere else. He just wanted everyone to leave her alone. But talking with him about her was so interesting. This was one of the big moments in our lives.

When Dean would mow the backyard, he would chase Nelson with the lawn mower, which had been a game for them ever since he was a puppy and tripped on his ears. While Dean would mow between the fence and the garage, he would always end up backing out, and Nelson always thought that it was a good time to get back. He would always poop behind Dean, which he then would step in. Dean would get so mad, but we had to laugh.

We saw Enid in the best of times and the worst of times. When the oil fields were producing and life was good in Enid, the population was around fifty thousand to almost sixty thousand. Then a bunch of the big businesses started to shut down or move. Champion Refinery moved to Texas somewhere, and Union Equity had shut its doors. The biggest employer left was Vance Air Force Base, and that was teetering on the line for closing. In fact, someone put a sign up at the Kansas-Oklahoma borderline: "Last one out of Enid, shut the light off." Crime went up, and the population dropped to thirty-five thousand. People were losing their homes, and banks were shutting down. In fact, Dean and I went through two closings. Some oil companies just locked their gates, and when their employees showed up for work, they found out that they didn't have a job anymore. But we managed. It wasn't ideal, but we came through, and Dean finally found a job at Bethany College.

I found out that you can never go back home, but we were stable again.

We didn't need a big house, and I was thinking that with the girls growing up, our pet days were over, until Jennifer found a kitten. We named him Tigger, and we now work for him. He is kind of a strange cat, but come to think of it, all our pets were strange. They say that their personalities come from the owners.

After Jennifer had moved out and Angie was going to be a senior, Tigger was acting real weird and started chasing Angie and I around the house. I grabbed the phone and called the vet. And he said it sounded like he had a fever. His instructions were to get the cat in a pillow case and bring him to the office. We were standing outside the house, and Tigger was looking at us through the window with his tongue out. I called Dean to come home and help us. He was so mad that we couldn't control the cat. I remember him saying under his breath, "It's just a cat."

He walked into the house, and as soon as Tigger saw him, he started chasing Dean around. But Dean did grab a pillowcase out of the cabinet. Somehow we got him in the pillowcase, and he had a high temperature and abscess. He had to stay a couple of nights with IVs, but you never expect to be chased out of your house by your cat. Tigger is alive and well; he is now thirteen years old and mostly has taken up our queen-size bed.

Dean stayed at Bethany College until he started having problems with his back. Both my brother and husband now have bad backs, and we are pretty sure it was from the oilfield. Asked now, they don't know how they survived.

MY BROTHER, GARY

We have had a lot of fun through the years and taken several trips, just the two of us. He has always been there for me through thick and thin, and as a nurse, he answered all the questions I would ask him, but now I try not to bother him; I want him as a brother and not a nurse. To this day, we will get to laughing about something that happened on the farm, and one of us has to leave the room because we couldn't quit.

Shortly after Dean and I were married and settled in Enid, Oklahoma, Gary and his wife, Linda, moved their children to Lindsey, Oklahoma, where they settled in Linda's grandmother's house, and Gary went to work for Otis, an oil field business. We saw each other, though not often. Dean and Gary's schedules were so different. But Gary's practical jokes were still alive and well.

When Mom had gotten real sick and they found out that her appendix had burst, she was in a lot of trouble. Gary picked me up in Enid and had gotten to Lindsborg. Dad was talking to the surgeon. Mom was having trouble waking up, and she would be in ICU for a couple of days. She also had a nasty infection from the appendix, and things just weren't good. We finally got Dad to go home around 2:00 a.m. so he could rest.

Gary and I had each a bed down in the basement, and I was so tired because mom was on my mind. I got ready for bed and shut the lights off. Gary was in the bathroom, and I had just gotten to sleep when Gary came in and said that something was wrong, and of course I pulled the light back on to see if I could help, and once my eyes were used to the light, there was Gary standing over me with white foam coming out of his mouth. He had put several Gas X tablets in his mouth to cause the foaming. But of course I screamed like I used to do, and once he stopped laughing we, heard those footsteps that we had heard several times before while growing up on the farm, and we knew we were in trouble. Dad yelled down the stairs at us like he used to. "Kids, stop whatever you were doing and go to bed." Dad didn't have a sense of humor at the time.

One Thanksgiving, we were all able to meet at Gary's, and Mom decided she wanted a family picture. Aunt Dorothy and Ernie were there, so Dorothy said she could take the picture, so this took awhile, getting our children to mind and look pleasant. They were all lined up, and all of a sudden there was a horrible smell that lofted through the group, and I thought Angie had pooped in her diaper. But it wasn't that, and finally the smell was so bad that we scattered in all directions.

Dorothy was ready and looked through the window of the camera and asked, "Where did everybody go?" By this time, we figured out who was literally behind the smell. The G.A.S. Man himself, Gary. Mom yelled at him as usual. "Gary Andrew Sundberg!" It's the way she used to say it. We told her it was Dad and her fault because of his initials. I found that picture from that fateful day. Our faces were either scared that Gary would have another go at it or Mom was on the warpath again.

When the jobs ran out in the oil field, Gary went to school for nursing, and Linda and Gary moved to Ellsworth, Kansas, after Dean and I and the girls moved back to Lindsborg. We were now closer.

He is a grandpa and loves all three of his grandchildren. We call each other or will meet in Lindsborg to spend time with Dad.

There are two more stories that I have saved for the last for a purpose. I think that these two stories are the best between Gary and I.

Gary, the Rubber Band Man

Gary is a great big brother, and we each got into our share of trouble. I always heard, "You know who's going to get hurt." And let me tell you, I was sick of hearing this all the time. This is one story that actually Mom learned the lesson. Gary was never mean to me; he was just the usual big brother.

Gary was around twelve at the time, so I had to be five. Flo and Oscar had sent a whole envelope full of rubber bands, which we never figured out why. But in the end, Mom sure wished that they hadn't.

It was the Saturday before Easter Sunday, and Mom was preparing the dinner for the next day since we always took turns between my grandparents and parents. Gary and I were setting the table with Mom's good dishes. She would set a place setting like she wanted it done, and then we would set the table. When we had finished, the weather wasn't at the best. Mom said that we could go find something else to do. We knew that if we didn't find something to do and we fought, she would find us a job. So Gary asked her if we could play with the rubber bands. She said yes without thinking this idea over. She had her mind on other things; she had just finished my Easter dress, and hers needed to be hemmed. My dress was a mint green with a cape of the same material to match with mint green strips. She bought new white shoes and socks with white gloves. The surprise was she also made a purse to match my outfit. I was going to look so coordinated.

We went up to Gary's room and decided to tie all the rubber bands together and see how far they would go. It took a long time, but we had fun and couldn't wait to see what was going to happen. I was just excited that Gary wanted to play with me.

When we finished, there was a long rope of rubber bands. Gary stayed upstairs in his room, and I took the other end downstairs and around the corner in the den. We would yell at each other how far it was going. I finally entered the hallway by the bathroom and almost past the refrigerator in the kitchen. I asked

Gary to stretch as far as it would go. Just as I went to show Mom, I heard something, and I looked back. The sound was from the staircase, coming around the corner in the den; then I saw it. *Wham, bam, snap!* I let out a scream, and Mom came around the corner and was shocked at the sight. Then Gary came from the staircase, kind of sheepish looking and breathing like he had been laughing until he saw me and stopped dead in his tracks.

The welts were already swelling, everywhere. Mom ran cold water in the bathtub and carefully put me in the tub, which hurt worse, and sat by me on the side of the tub and kept running water over me and thought that might help. The welts were all over my face, arms, neck, stomach, legs, ankles, and everywhere in between. I saw Mom thinking about how my Easter outfit would look on me now. She put so much cold paste that I was shivering and all this with my clothes still on. I was still crying pretty hard, and being in the bathroom, it echoed. Dad came in for afternoon coffee and heard all the commotion and came in before washing up in the washroom. Gary knew he was in trouble then. So, in the end, Gary got spanked. Easter morning was a flop for me. Gary still got to hunt for Easter eggs but shared them without being asked, and he kept telling me he was sorry even when he didn't have to. I laid over a sheet on the couch with some really nasty welts. I wasn't able to wear my new outfit, and I missed going to Sunday school and church, but that wasn't a big loss. Mom ended up staying home with me and got the dinner ready for our guests.

Grandma felt so bad that she played a song on the piano for me. The piano was hers, but they couldn't get it moved to their house and left it at our house. There was one song that she used to play; I wish I could hear her play it again. Dad said that none of us knew what kind of damage the rubber bands could do. Mom really thanked her parents. We would communicate by tape; we could hear everyone's voices and send them back and forth through the mail.

We laugh about it now, but back then it wasn't funny, and then I knew I would have to do something to get back a Gary, and this is where the trouble would start.

The Snicker Doodle Story

Once Mom had taught me to bake, I was a baking fool. I loved making cookies, and this is when we hand mixed them and used a bunch of baking supplies like flour, butter, baking soda, etc. Snicker doodles are cookies that you mix up and refrigerate for twenty-four hours before baking.

Mom and Dad were going away for the evening, and Gary and I were staying home. I had asked if I could bake my cookies while they were gone. It was only one recipe, and it would go fast. They said yes.

When baking snicker doodles, you roll the dough into balls and roll them into sugar. Gary used to like to throw things up in the air and catch them with his mouth. This was during the winter months when things weren't as busy for Dad, and Mom wanted the ceiling in the living and dining room lowered, and they had done some remolding while working on the ceiling. Dad knew that he could do the ceiling, and they had picked out some beautiful white tile.

Gary bet me that he could throw three balls of dough in the air and catch them in his mouth, so the bet was on. Do you see anything wrong with this bet?

He threw the first two dough balls and caught them, and then he threw the last ball. We were in the living room, and up the dough went, and Gary stood looking up at the ceiling, waiting to catch the dough, but it never came back. It had stuck to Dad's new ceiling tile. Remember, it was white.

I thought that I had been had until I went to the living room and saw Gary's face. It was as white as the tile. Then I looked up, and I bet you could imagine how our faces looked. I won the bet, but now we had to clean the ceiling off. Gary got the kitchen stool and cleaned the dough off, but the grease spot was still there. We got rags and wet washcloths and started working on the spot. We tried everything from soap and water to toothpaste. Nothing worked, so we got Mom's hair dryer down and took the hood off the end and I plugged it in. There was Gary, standing on the stool with the hair dryer hanging over his shoulder like a purse, drying the ceiling. We had bought the hair dryer for Mom for Christmas, and she was so tickled that she could dry her hair and walk around in the kitchen with the machine over her shoulder.

We kept asking each other if we could see the spot. Finally, we both agreed that there was no way anyone could see it. This was our second mistake.

Gary helped me finish up baking the cookies and cleaning up. Then we packed them in the freezer and then sat and waited for our parents to come home. They got there, and we were ready to go to bed. Up the stairs we went, and as we got to the top, Mom yelled up the stairs and said that dad wanted to ask us something. We knew we had been caught.

Going back downstairs had to be one of the longest walks ever. We got to the kitchen, and Dad was sitting at the table where he had carried the phone from the living room, but the lights were out, and we thought there was hope. He hung the phone up, and all he had to do was point his finger up as he turned on the light on to put the phone back in its place. They gave us a chance to explain what happened and then told us to go to bed and that we would discuss it in the morning.

The morning came, and while we were eating breakfast, there was a list of extra chores to pick from, but the first thing that was always done was to make our beds and clean up our rooms. While Gary and I were doing our jobs, we heard our parents laughing through the heating vents that were in both our rooms, but we thought it was wise not to say anything.

Dad replaced the ceiling tile, and I don't think Gary ever ate another snicker doodle again.

A LOVE STORY

I am sure that everyone remembers the movie *Love Story* that came out in the early seventies. *Love Story* has nothing on my parents. I admit it wasn't always perfect, but I don't really remember them fighting, at least not in front of us. They always said that they discussed problems, and their grandchildren always said that they fought "funny." I do remember one time when Dad was reading the paper at the kitchen table and Mom was washing dishes and discussing something with him, and he wasn't paying attention to her. She then went over to him and ripped the newspaper in half and asked if she had his attention then.

My parents were married for fifty-nine years. When thcy both retired, they spent every day together. From walking two miles a day to traveling, they were always together.

For their fortieth anniversary, Gary's family and my family gave them a reception at the church, and as I said, they never had a big wedding, so we asked them if they would like to renew their wedding vows. They thought that would be okay, so thirty minutes before the reception started, Pastor Molander stood up and announced that they had decided to renew their vows in front of everyone. It just so happened to be a perfect time because almost all were there to watch, but the difference was Gary and I stood up with them, and Mom had a bouquet of flowers that she always wanted.

As the service started, I don't think there was a dry eye in the place, but when the pastor asked Dad if his wedding band was the same one that he received on their wedding day, his remark was, "No, the first ring wore out." Everybody went from crying to laughing. Gary and I couldn't even look at each other without laughing at the way Dad said it. Anyway, Mom got her wedding, and the reception went so well with their family and friends around them. Of course, we even had a wedding cake for them.

The other night, I sat at Dad's apartment and looked at their photo albums of all the trips they got to take together. They went to Sweden, many cruises, and traveled the United States, and there was one trip that Gary and I tried to get them not to go. Two weeks after 9–11, they went on a cruise, and we really didn't want them to go. They had a chance to have their money refunded if people were uneasy about leaving the country at that time. Well, everything went fine until they docked at Boston. Then the security had just started at the Boston airport, and I think they even missed their plane, or something had happened. But they wouldn't admit that it was a little too much.

They also liked taking the trips through the bank, and all the people that went knew each other. They really enjoyed those trips.

When they were home, they had their certain routine every day: breakfast and reading the paper, then a two-mile walk, back home, do a few things, lunch, and this is when they had their big meal for the day. Then in the afternoon they would rest because Mom was supposed to rest with her RA as the years went on. Then they always attended events that went on in Lindsborg and around the area. They used to go dancing on Wednesday nights before Mom got to where she couldn't dance anymore. We never knew where they were, but they always seemed to have a good time. I know now that everyone comments on how odd it seems that they're not together. They used to go to exercise at the hospital, and now Dad has continued the same. We always said they were in a rut, but what a nice rut.

Their fiftieth anniversary was going to be a big party, and a week before is when we found out that Dad had cancer in the bone of his leg, and they had to put a steel rod in his leg. Then the next day, dad had a stroke. So everyone—brothers, sisters, their children, and their grandchildren—had cake and ice cream at the rehabilitation hospital. The hospital even let us decorate and provided the plates. Dad was in a wheelchair and seemed to enjoy the party, but in the pictures that were taken, he looked awfully gray. But he recovered, and he took radiation treatments and made it through; it's been ten years now.

When we had Christmas in 2004, Gary and I were sitting at the table watching everyone open their presents. As I was looking at Mom, I gasped at how much she had deteriorated through the year. Gary then warned me that the next year was going to be rough. I kind of knew what he was talking about, but I wasn't ready and put it out of my mind. He was right.

Mom's RA had started to cause problems with her heart. The prognosis wasn't good. Gary and I started to go with them when they saw her specialists. Gary finally had talked to Dad about her health problems and that this was not good and that drugs weren't going to help her anymore.

The next thing we knew, in March 2005, they bought a beautiful home and sold their condo, and then we got confused about what was going on. We were giving Mom a birthday party and they announced their plans. They moved in the middle of April. We knew there was something behind this. April came, and Mom said her leg was hurting and was admitted to the hospital with blood clots. The whole family got together, and it was one, two, three, shift. They had everything boxed up already. Thanks to Linda, my sister-in-law; she helped me with the kitchen the night before, and I couldn't have done it without her help. We both had been around Mom enough to know how she liked things, and we wanted her to come home with everything put away, furniture arranged in its place, as if nothing else had changed. The moving went well, except we bounced the pie cabinet out the back of the truck, but Gary is so handy; he fixed it back up, and you could hardy believe it happened. Angie and her sorority sisters helped by cleaning the condo that afternoon and by 2:00 p.m., Dad and I went to visit Mom at the hospital and told her everything was done. She was teased that she didn't want to do the moving part, but we all knew how it was.

She loved that house; it had large glass windows for sunlight, and I told her that there were still about ten boxes left in the garage, and she didn't seem to worry about it.

She enjoyed seeing Angie's senior art exhibit and graduation the next day from Bethany College, but Mom had a health issue at the graduation. Luckily Dean had his keys with him, and we were able to unlock the elevator and helped her to the car. We had Angie's reception at their house, and it was a great house to have company. We kept Mom in a chair to where we didn't let her up. It was a beautiful day, and people were outside and inside.

The next occasion was Angie and Dirk's wedding. At the first of the year, Angie, Jennifer, Mom, and I went shopping for Angie's wedding dress and bought one. What we were interested in was Jennifer. By the time of the wedding, she would be three weeks away from her due date.

Jennifer gave Angie a shower, and it was a great shower, but when Mom was getting out of the car, she fell and broke her gift. I went out and helped her in the building, and she was so upset. I remember her asking me then what was happening to her.

July was the wedding at Bethany Lutheran

Church, and the rehearsal went well, but the day of the wedding, Mom was not good and ended up sitting in the wing of the church instead of with us. We had most the pictures taken before the service, and you can see that we were holding her up very carefully because if you would grab her to hold on, her skin was starting to tear; it was so thin.

The photographer was great, and I knew his son from the college. I asked them if he could take a picture of Mom for me when she didn't know it. I explained why, and I have a beautiful picture of her now. It was one of the last pictures.

The reception was held at a banquet room at a hotel in Salina, and Mom came, but when the dancing started, Dad and my uncle Duke decided she had a big day, so they took her home. Boy, was she mad; she wanted to watch the kids dance.

The next day, both sides of the family watched Dirk and Angie open their gifts at Mom and Dad's. Angie wanted her grandparents to see what they got. Everyone was exhausted; Mary (Dirk's mother) and I have become good friends. Mom had made the comment about not seeing Angie too much the last two years; she called her "the Shadow." Now, Angie had a job in town and was able to see her grandparents every night after the wedding.

Jennifer made it through the wedding and had Lucas two weeks later. Dad brought Mom down to see the new baby, but she was pretty weak. Howard helped her hold the baby. This was the last time she was at our house.

October started her decline. The town was celebrating Svensk Hyllingsfest festival, and Dean needed to be at work early, so we were on the road by five thirty, plenty of time to help Mom. I rented a wheelchair from the pharmacy, but we had a flat tire and were really late getting to town. The parade started at 10:00 a.m., but we always got to our places in front of the church an hour earlier. I didn't get Mom's makeup or her hair curled before the parade, and I was really upset that I had let her down, but she seemed to enjoy the parade. They were invited to a brunch afterward, so I put her in her rocker and went to work, and she looked really nice to go out. Gary and Linda brought their grandsons with them, and after Mom and Dad left, we talked about the trip that Gary and Linda were going on by themselves to the East Coast. They were driving and were planning to leave early the following week. They planned to be gone for two weeks, but our lives sure did change while they were gone.

The Saturday morning after the Hyllningsfest, Dad called and said Mom wasn't good. So we jumped in the car, and Angie beat us to their house. I walked in and went straight to their bedroom and was shocked at how mom looked. If you would touch her, she would scream. I felt her pulse, and it was very weak. I picked up the phone and called 911. This was the time when Mom started to go downhill. She was admitted to the hospital, and I called Gary. I called just to tell him, not for them to come home. I called Mom and Dad everyday from then on.

Dean and I came the following Saturday, and everything seemed fine, so we took Dad out for lunch.

We were back within the hour, and the doctor and nurses were all over. Mom was hemorrhaging, and her veins weren't good enough for a large needle for blood. They decided to transfer her to Salina. When they carried her out, I made them stop to say we would be there and I loved her. Dad then said something, and they were off. We arrived, and they told us to go to the ICU. Angie, Dirk, and LaShae, Gary's daughter, were waiting, and they told me to get in there, so I walked in and found Mom's room.

They had the needle in her neck, and she was hooked to everything. I turned around and got Dad. Boy, I wished I never been there when my parents saw each other. I heard Mom say that she thought she was going to die before she got to Salina.

LaShae called Gary and gave the number to the nurses' desk so he could talk to them. Then he wanted to talk to me and said they would be on the road within the hour. I was glad to hear that piece of news.

Angie and Dirk took Dad to their home; they had just moved to Salina. Dean and I slept in the waiting room, and I told Mom's nurse to come and get me if she needed me, and she did. We heard Angie say not to worry; they had everything he needed, even "poop powder." She took such good care of him; she even tucked him into bed.

Mom was thrashing around, and I leaned over the bed and held her and told her I was there; I wasn't leaving. I said that her monitors were looking better, and her color was better. Then I sang a song she used to sing to me when I was sick, and I petted her hair. After a couple hours, she settled down, and I went back to the waiting room and collapsed. I was woken up by the smell of fresh coffee. There was a hot ICU cup of coffee. I found out later that it was Mom's nurse saying thank you for the help.

Howard, Jennifer, and the boys came first, and Jennifer went in to see her by herself. By the time she came back, Angie had brought Dad back, so he went in and found out they had moved a recliner in her room. So we left them alone, and we started putting puzzles together, and they had a bunch. Eventually, everyone had gotten there, and they gave our family a room with a table, chairs, TV, and whatever else we needed. Everyone got to go see her one at a time while Dad was there. Then their friends started coming up and bringing cookies and other treats. Dad made sure everyone ate in the cafeteria.

When I saw Gary and Linda through the window, I wanted to cry, but I didn't. I worried about them coming too. They went right in. Gary said he was afraid that he wouldn't get here in time.

They found out where she was bleeding from, and there were two nights they told us Mom wasn't going to make it through the night. Finally, they stepped her down and out of ICU. But her heart started going haywire, and they had to start her heart again and put her back in the ICU. Finally, we talked the doctor into bringing her back to the hospital in Lindsborg; it would have been closer for everyone. Howard would come on his lunch hour, and Dean would come up when he was done with work. They said she could go to the hospital in Lindsborg. I hated that she had come home to die.

Dad started staying at the hospital; they had a pullout bed. We had her in a family room. Then Dad would leave and hurry back; he made sure he was there to feed her, and if we were home, we would take over to help him. Every night, Angie would pop in and see them and watch *Wheel of Fortune.* I told you they were in a rut.

When Mom was bad, and Dean was making me go home to rest, I asked God if I could have a little more time. I remember I wrote it out on a sheet of paper. He gave me eight more weeks, but the last week, I felt guilty because she was in so much pain. But we had some good times talking about how my parents met, and then her fingernails started to grow out beautifully, so I would shape them and polish them for her. That just thrilled her.

She wanted to go home for a half a day, so Gary carried her in with all her tubes, and I fixed her oyster soup; that was her favorite. She didn't eat very much, but from her recliner she could see me and watched me while I was cleaning up the kitchen. Gary put her in their bed, and she stayed there the rest of the day. Gary, Dad, and I took her back to the hospital. Gary leaned over and gave her a kiss good-bye and said he would see her in two days. She looked at Dad and said, "I must be dying; he never wants me to kiss him; he always squirms away."

She had wanted to be cremated, but we all told her we couldn't do it, and she decided that a casket was fine as long as just the family saw her and no one else. We agreed.

The following Sunday was Christmas, and I had bought her a purple lounging outfit with a cardinal on the front, and the nurse said that she and I would give her a sponge bath. I was so shocked at her little body. Mom was way under a hundred pounds, and she had bedsores. It was horrible, but I didn't let on. We got her new outfit on, and it really looked nice. Then she asked me to take her for a ride in the wheelchair, and it was just beautiful outside for that time of the year. We had our girl talk, which was great, and she enjoyed going outside. I took her back to her room; she was ready to rest before lunch, so I put my head down on her bed. A while later, I felt somebody running her fingers through my hair, and as I opened my eyes, I saw it was Mom doing what she used to do when I was sick. She was comforting me.

I fed her, and then she wanted to take a nap, so Gary and Dean said lunch was ready at the house. Everyone was there; Gary and my kids, great-grandchildren, and Dad really enjoyed the afternoon.

We went back to see her, and Dad wanted to give her supper. She wasn't good, and they gave her more pain medication; she didn't eat supper. We left Dad, but I told him I'd be back in a couple of hours. At about 3:00 a.m. I opened the door very quietly and saw Dad sitting in the recliner by her bed, holding her hand, and when he looked up, I showed him I brought an apple and a knife to share with him. He had done this right before they put her in the family room. So

I cut the apple up and we shared it. We didn't have to say a thing to each other.

December 26, 2005, was horrible for Mom; they couldn't get the pain controlled, so hospice brought some medicine to make her relax. Before they got there, I held her in my arms, and she told me that she wanted her mother. I replied that I wanted my mom. Those blue eyes looked right through me. I then said a thank you for adopting me. We both shared a few tears. She didn't want me there when she died.

Angie, Dad, and I, were never able to talk with her again. Angie went on home, and I stayed with Dad. Mom was out from the pain medication, and she would stop breathing, and the nurses started to watch the clock. Every two hours we would turn her from side to side. Finally, I couldn't watch any more, and one of the nurses told me to go onto the house. I was sitting in the dark, and it was around 6:30 a.m. and the phone rang.

A Final Good-Bye

My dad was on the other end telling me to come, and Dean had me there within minutes. Before we left, I called the hospital to find out which way to get in. They said the front doors are always unlocked at six a.m. Dean dropped me off in the front, and I ran to the door that was supposed to be open; it wasn't. I ran straight into it and bounced off. So I tried again, and it happened again. Finally, I started banging on the door, yelling. Finally, the nurse saw me and came running. She opened the door, and I ran to where my parents were, but one was gone.

I remember looking at her and thinking that I needed to thank someone for letting me have eight weeks longer, and I did and asked please take care of her.

After Gary and Linda got there, I let the nurse call the funeral home. Gary took Dad back to the house, and Linda and I stayed. We cleaned up the room and took her Christmas tree down, and there was a knock on the door and it was the funeral home. We left and went home too. As I got to the door, there was Jennifer, and I fell into her arms. Dean had gone back to the house and called the girls with the news. Angie got there soon after. I was walking around, not putting anything away. The girls had moved our suitcases into the guest room so Dad could have his room back. Then I found the outfit that Mom wore to Angie's wedding and picked out her jewelry and a white stuffed bear that the grandchildren had bought her.

The days went on very slowly after the funeral, and I was lucky that we could stay with Dad four days out of the week, and then Gary would come and see him. We needed a project to work on and decided to unpack the boxes that were left in the garage. We thought it was mostly junk until we found all of Mom's scrapbooks that she had kept through the years. One book was all about their wedding and where they stayed. Another one was about December 7, 1941; she kept all the news clippings and a lot of things that are historical now. The next book, I picked it up to open it, and a clipping fell out and looking at it shocked me. It was a clipping of a house design that she had cut out of the paper, and at the bottom was written "my dream house." I want to tell you that it wasn't too far off the mark of the house we were standing in. We really enjoyed looking at them, and I found out that my mother had been a girl, lady, a girlfriend, a wife, and a mother; she had a life before us.

Dad and I went to Salina for something, and on the way home, Dad told me that he didn't want to stay in the new house any longer than he had to; they were not together long enough for it to be theirs. Then I found out that Mom had found out that it was for sale, and she knew who lived there and had been in the house, so Dad bought the house for her, thinking that he might have a little longer. Three months later, the house sold, and he moved into a two-bedroom apartment.

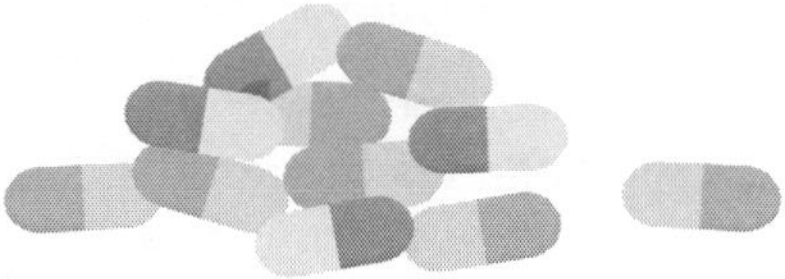

A CARDINAL STORY

Mom loved watching the birds from the kitchen, and red cardinals were her favorite. This story is so fantastic, but there are several people who witnessed this bird.

A few weeks after Mom had passed, I noticed this red cardinal sitting on their outdoor furniture. He would cock his head, like he knew I was there. A couple of days later, that stupid bird started ramming his body into the patio door; then he would start pecking on the glass for quite a while, and this went on every day. Angie still came over and watched *Wheel of Fortune* with Dad. He always walked Angie to her car, and she started noticing a bird was pooping on her car, and he always made sure he hit her mirror on the side of the car. We thought this was kind of funny. Then I saw that cardinal sitting on the brick windowsill, watching Dad working in the kitchen, and the bird was very attentive.

Gary came over and parked his car next to Dad's car in the driveway. Guess which car the bird hit? It wasn't Dad's. Then the bird was watching at the patio door. Dad went in their bedroom to put something away, and I noticed he forgot something, so I started to go to where he was, and I saw that the bird was gone. As I got into the bedroom, I saw that bird sitting on the bedroom patio and watching Dad.

Everyone that came over left with birdie poop on his or her car. I was taking the trash out when that stupid bird tried to dive bomb me; I didn't make it to the trash. I went and got Dean. He said that I was trying to get out of emptying the trash; he was teasing. When he came back in, the bird aimed and fired and pooped on Dean's head, and it was runny. He immediately washed his hair several times while I laughed. Dad never noticed what the bird was doing to us. He had other things on his mind.

Gary came over the next day, and I told him what happened to Dean, and he wondered if he should carry an umbrella. Gary laughed so hard, and it actually was kind of funny. His comment was that Mom came back as a red cardinal and was still peeking at everyone, trying to tell us what needs to be done. I thought he hit the nail on the head.

Moving day came, and it was all on our minds if that red cardinal would follow Dad over to his new apartment. The answer is no! This little red cardinal sure did lighten things up at a time that we all needed it.

My Dad Today

Our dad is doing very well these days for almost ninety years young. He stays very busy with playing cards several times a week. He's on the board for the senior center, the American Legion, and every Memorial Day he announces the names of the veterans who died during the year and also pays tribute to the veterans of all wars who died in action from Lindsborg and surrounding areas. He still "roars" with the Lyons Club, and he has found new friends while attending hospice on Wednesday mornings. Of course, there's church on Sundays, and he still participates with the club that he and Mom belonged to. He eats a few times at the senior center, loves cooking oatmeal, and learned to bake the cookies that you just put on the cookie sheet. He continues walking at the work out center at the hospital. He took me to the orthopedic surgeon when I broke both of my feet and was there with Dean standing by my bed when I woke from the surgeries and has helped Gary with different projects.

We worried before and after Mom passed that this might be one of those cases where the husband dies shortly after his wife of a broken heart.

I do remember the first time he drove to Newton for lunch and spent an afternoon with all of us. I was outside waiting for him, and as he drove up, Mom wasn't sitting in the front seat like she always did. I remarked to him that she should have been with him. All he said was, "I know." Like he says, he still is wearing a wedding ring, so he is still married to her.

Gary and I love him very much and probably don't tell him enough, and we still don't know how he found out about the buckets in "The Bucket Story."

A FEW OF MY FRIENDS

I have had lots of individuals in my life, and it was hard to know whom to write about. These are the ones I picked.

Cancer and the Man Who Saved My Life

Sometimes it's very strange how things come about, like if it hadn't been so hot and I hadn't wore white shorts at that time; I didn't wear shorts in public. Or I was seeing a doctor before my appointment with the dermatologist and he wanted me to show him a mole on the back of my leg at my next appointment. Or I had an hour to wait, so Dean and I went to the Q-shop for something to drink, and I mentioned to Dean that maybe I have the Big C.

This actually happened and in order. I was seeing Dr. Kelley, a dermatologist for something that medications do to your skin; he was taking a couple of stitches out. I stood up, and he asked if he could look at the mole on the back of my leg. The clock started ticking.

His reaction was totally scary. The first question was "Where did that come from?" because he didn't notice it before. I had jeans on, and I only had my shirt off for the biopsy. Then he looked straight at me and said I had cancer, melanoma cancer to be exact. He wanted a biopsy right then, and everyone was excited and I had just seen my life pass before me. His nurse at the time had loaded a syringe to deaden the area. The nurse had forgotten to lock the syringe, and as Dr. K injected the drugs, the liquid squirted in his eyes. He started washing his eyes out, and I felt so bad because that really had to hurt. She asked him if it would deaden his eyes. He asked her, "What do you think?" Finally, the biopsy was done, and it would be back at the end of the week. I remember asking if he wanted a ride home; stupid, huh? He had taken the middle out, and we would wait almost two weeks before he would do the surgery. We asked why, and he said he had disturbed the mole and wanted it to heal. The stitches would come out. Then we would set a date for the surgery. I cried all the way home, and Dean didn't know what to say.

I thought that I had won the biggest fight of my life a few years a go, and now I had cancer. Mom always told me, "God doesn't give you any more than you can handle." Well, I sure wanted to discuss a few things with him. Mom and Dad were in San Jose, California, visiting her brother, and Dad was over his treatments for his cancer. So I called Gary; he couldn't believe what he was hearing. He said that the mole had been there since he could remember; I had always had it. Could the doctor be wrong? (I hoped.) Then we told the girls, and I started to cry again. At that point, I wanted to take a steak knife and remove it myself. I wanted it out of my system. I told Mom over the phone, and I don't think it connected until she got home, and the surgery was the following Monday.

I then needed someone to talk to. I was scared, and Dean's mother was no help. The doctor put her in the hospital because she thought that she had cancer in her face, and he wanted her out of our hair. Don't ask.

I called my second mother, Lois Ferm, and Emma Sunderberg, my cousin that lived across the road most of my life. Both of them really settled me down, and I don't remember what they said. Thank God I thought of them. Life was pretty horrible until Jennifer and Howard came from Houston for a long weekend. Everyone decided they wanted to talk with Dr. Kelley.

I remember wondering if I was going to see my grandchildren or if I would get to see Angie graduate, questions that had no answers.

Dr. Kelley took out the stitches and read the biopsy. Positive for melanoma cancer; he was right on the mark. We all went into another room to talk. He wasn't sure yet about having chemotherapy, radiation, or both. He told them that ten years ago they would have taken my leg off, but there was a different type of surgery, and he drew out what the incision would look like. Their questions had been answered, and the surgery was set.

Back in the car, everyone was very quiet, and we drove around Hutchinson. I don't remember who said it, but I know it had to be one of the girls. The doctor was blond, blue eyes, and very handsome, just look at him; I wouldn't need anesthesia. The guys said that he looked like a lot of other doctors, and to be honest, I hadn't noticed until I saw him for the surgery. Boy, did that lighten the mood.

Mom and Dad got home and really wanted to go with us for the surgery, but we didn't know how long it would be.

He numbed my whole leg and started in. We talked, and he said he went pretty deep. After he took enough tissue and the mole, each layer had to be stitched, and the top layer stitches would be removed in ten days.

I didn't want to look, and the pain came on before we got home. The dressing had to be changed two times a day, and Mom, Dad, and Dean handled everything. We did exactly what he wrote down for directions. Mom fixed up a box with all the supplies and several tubes of antibiotic. The second day of changing the bandage, I saw what the incision looked like, and it shocked me how it looked. I remember when my parents saw it; it shocked them too.

Dean and Angie wouldn't let me do much but go to the bathroom and lie in bed and watch TV. Friends brought casseroles over, and of course, my parents were there frequently.

At the next appointment, the stitches came out, and the doctor couldn't believe how I was healing, and they got the biopsy back; no treatments necessary. But I had checkups for a month, three months, six months, and finally a year. I remember looking at the mole in the biopsy cup, and it was a lot bigger under the skin, and by following his complete instructions, you can hardly see a scar. He did a beautiful job.

I was always so scared for each appointment, but now it's like seeing a good friend. But you do not miss an appointment, and if I find something to question, I call him, and he makes time for me. On a visit shortly after the surgery, as a joke, Dean brought him a pair of goggles, just in case that problem happened again. My cancer surgery was in 1997.

Melanoma Cancer

What do Troy Aikman, Sam Donaldson, and John McCain have in common? They are survivors of melanoma cancer.

In 1930, melanoma was almost unheard of but due to the changes in the ultraviolet light from the sun, is more common. The problem with melanoma is that it is very tricky and unpredictable cancer that can silently metastasize to the lungs and the brain (common targets) years, even decades, after the original tumor is excised from the skin. The absolute key is prevention.

Worldwide, it annually strikes an estimated 132,000 people, with an estimated 48,000 deaths. This means one in thirty-two if the last year doesn't show a different from the American Cancer Society. Australia and New Zealand have the highest melanoma rates on the planet. One in twenty-five will get melanoma.

The public heath department has taken measures to fight the disease. They have a "No Hat, No Play" rule. Every child must wear a hat to play outside. Recess times are often rescheduled outside the 11:00 a.m. to 3:00 p.m. time frame. Soccer games played without hats under the high sun in the U.S. are delayed until a safer time. Children are also wearing neck to knee swimsuit on beaches and at the pools. Many pools and playgrounds are now covered by expansive tents or newly planted trees.

There are many misleading claims of sunscreen manufacturers, so the FDA has cracked down on the confusing terms such as sunblock, waterproof, all-day protection, and visible and/or infrared light protection.

Remember, have a dermatologist check out anything on your skin, attend all checkups afterward, and wear a hat with a wide brim to cover your head, face, neck, and ears. Avoid with the sun between 10:00 a.m. and 4:00 p.m. Sit under an umbrella or shading. It's time to get your children to wear a hat while playing outside. This is not all the information about melanoma; go on the Internet and read as much as you can get your hands on or get in touch with the American Cancer Society.

Maureen Reagan, daughter of the late President Ronald Reagan, Bob Marley, and Eva Cassidy, a rising folk musician star, and recently, we heard a member Bruce Springsteen's E Street band were lost to melanoma cancer. These famous people lost the battle. Cancer of any kind doesn't care if you're rich or poor.

To Dr. Russell Kelley: Thank you so much for everything. I'm not sure. How do you thank some one for saving your life?

Duck Soup, an Unforgettable Character

My aunts and uncles all had and have very loving qualities, but this is a story about my uncle Duke. He was my mother's only brother, whom she loved very much and usually would shake her head at because of the stuff he use to get by with.

Duck Soup was a name my grandpa Oscar, his father, had for him, and if you want to get his goat, I dare you to call him that.

I didn't get to see my uncle very much while growing up, but the times we were together were unforgettable. I'm proud to say that I'm his one and only niece, and he is my godfather.

The first thing that I remember him for is a letter that he wrote me about my missing toe. He wrote that my toe started growing back. But it kept growing, and Mom ended up cutting a hole in the shoe so my toe could grow through the hole. This story went on, and I still have it in my scrapbook. I think he must have had too much time on his hands, but I knew it was written with love.

When my parents and I were in California visiting my mom's relatives, there was a family reunion at the Russian River. My mom's aunt had a vacation getaway built on the side of the hill. All the bedrooms were on the lower level, which was still high off from the driveway. They had a pulley and rope to pull your luggage up with. The upstairs had a wonderful large room where we met in the mornings and ate, and we would sit by their wood stove at night to ward the chill off or play cards at a large table. This was a neat cabin. One night, Duke was teaching me to play poker, which I had never learned before. He took me for all my allowance, plus the money I had saved up for the trip and wouldn't give it back. He made me cry, and of course, he has never forgotten it. I now have turned the tables on him and tell him how horrible he was to take my money. We would swim in the Russian River during the day and would race across. At that time, it wasn't very deep. He brings that time up usually every time we talk.

In 1967, we planned a family road trip since Gary had graduated from high school, and my folks thought that it would be the last trip with just us. The trip was planned around a wedding of my mom's cousin in San Francisco. Dad had bought a new car, and Gary and I weren't quite over aggravating each other, so I ended up on the floor of the car so he could sleep, and the hump in the middle wasn't that comfortable for a new car. Duke had relocated to Albuquerque, New Mexico, with his job and had a new home that he shared with his wife and Harvey. Gary thought his front lawn was neat and volunteered to mow it any time since it was all rock, no grass. The pool was really neat, and a good time was had by all. Duke showed me where I was sleeping, and this is where I fell in love with Harvey. Duke had won him at the fair for fifty cents; being six feet tall with twelve-inch feet, pink with a tie, and wearing a hat with two holes for his ears, I fell for him. I slept on top of him instead of the bed and sat on him while everyone was playing cards. But it came time to push on and our good-byes were said.

Duke and his wife, Leo, met us in San Francisco for the wedding, and Mom made me a pink lace dress with a pink ribbon tie on the front; I felt elegant. Watching everyone dance and drink champagne was new for me. But one of the biggest moments in my life was my first dance, a time that every girl remembers. Duke could really "cut a rug," as they used to say. This was the fanciest wedding I had ever been to, and I remember it to this day. I remember the cake topper was so beautiful, and I got to borrow it for my wedding.

This trip was a once-in-a-lifetime trip in Victorville, California. We visited the Roy Roger and Dale Evans Museum in Apple Valley and saw the original Trigger, stuffed. I also saw a real roadrunner in the desert, like the Looney Toons cartoons. Sea World, Disneyland, downtown Hollywood were an experience. Duke took me down the most crooked street in the world, and I rode the cable cars all the way down to Fisherman's Wharf. We ended up our trip at my grandparents' new home where they were going to retire, and we swam in their new pool. Clear Lake Highlands was a really nice, neat little town to the north of San Francisco. I ended up with a horrible ear infection, and Mom took me to a doctor. But it still was a great trip, and I got to know Duke better.

The following Christmas, everybody came for the holidays, and our house was full to the brim. A few days before, I wasn't feeling good and ended up with strep throat. I still had the temperature, and everyone was keeping a close eye on me. Dad moved me downstairs in the den where he had made up the couch. I don't think I ate Christmas dinner or opened presents, but Duke and Leo came on the twenty-fourth, and everybody wanted me to see their car when they drove up. Harvey was sitting in his seat with the seatbelt on, and when Duke brought him in to me, I wanted him to have the couch, and I would sleep on the floor, but that didn't last long. That rabbit was a permanent resident on my bed until I got married and moved away. I know there were times I had to sew him up, and I would suppose he must have been dirty but too big to throw in the washer. I loved him. I was glad that Duke was there, our first Christmas and last Christmas together.

Our relationship went on through the years and all the crazy stuff. Duke was never a father, but probably would have made a great one. We wrote to each other and probably his greatest practical joke was on my wedding day. They couldn't come because my aunt was very sick, and Duke thought it was better they stayed at home. But it all started with a phone call that morning and my parents and Flo and Oscar were sitting around the kitchen table having coffee. I answered the phone, and the voice asked if I was Wendy, and I said, "Speaking." The voice at the other end said that he was visiting relatives, and they thought that I might show him around. I told him that I was sorry but thought I could find someone else for him. He said no, and then we talked for a while. He then asked if I was busy that night and would I like to go out with him. I said no and that I was busy, and then he wanted to know what I was doing and could he possibly tag along with me. I didn't recognize his voice but noticed that everybody in the kitchen was laughing, but Oscar probably told one of his famous jokes.

This conversation wasn't over yet. I told him at 6:00 p.m. I was getting married, and I didn't really think he should be there since I didn't know him and frankly didn't care. He would not take no for an answer, and finally he asked me why I was marrying Dean and said I was too young and how did I know he was the right one, and on and on. I got mad then and started yelling into the phone when all of a sudden I heard his voice and, of course, he was laughing. I thought it was a dirty trick but loved him anyway. Boy, was I gullible, but I had other things on my mind. I told Dean about the conversation later that evening. He laughed about it too. Duke's joke became a classic through the years.

Whenever we called each other, Dean and Mom both agreed that listening to the conversation was better then talking. Believe me when I say nothing was sacred.

When we were getting ready for Angie's wedding in July of 2005, I called Duke and Virginia (Duke's second wife) and asked them to come and then told Duke about Mom and her condition. They came, and Dad, Mom, and I met them at the airport. I had Mom in a wheelchair, and Duke was absolutely shocked. He had to go outside while we were waiting for their luggage. They came again for Thanksgiving when she was in the hospital. Duke and I talked about if he would be coming back when Mom died, and he told me to call him no matter what time, and he didn't think he would come back. Well, less than a month later, I had to make that call, and I thought about how Duke was the last one in Mom's family, but we were still his family, and he still is my godfather, and our love for each other hasn't wavered.

Remember the famous song that Nat King Cole sang, "Unforgettable"? I will always think of him when this song is played

What a Friend I Have in Linda

I met Linda while working at Bethany College in the cafeteria, and as soon as we met, I knew we would be friends and something extraordinary was ahead of us.

The first time we wanted our husbands to meet, I had them over for supper and found out they liked the same things: football, KU basketball, the Chiefs, cards, and just about any old thing. Our husbands got along really well, but they knew they had something in common: us. They always just shook their heads at us.

There were a lot of adventures ahead of us, like the time when we got to laughing and started snorting. Although while laughing, she sneezed and Jell-O came out her nose. Then we laughed harder. We were made for each other.

Poor thing, she had acid reflux so bad that I started carrying Lifesavers, and when she would start coughing, I gave her one and headed off the trouble. We were in a secondhand store when I heard her start the cough, and I threw the pack of Lifesavers across the store to her. Boy, did I get the stares.

Have you ever gone to a garage sale and ever gotten a traffic ticket? We did. We loved to go to garage sales, and we would find one and drive by to see if there was something interesting, and this time we saw something. Linda hit the brakes and parked the wrong way. We weren't gone long and didn't even buy anything, and as we got back to her car, there was a ticket between the windshield and the wipers. We couldn't believe it, so we went right up to the police station and split the amount in half. There went our garage sale money. We always set aside a set amount to spend, and I'm telling you, she could smell the best garage sales out. We used to go to the college games together, football and basketball, and we always got into trouble at the Sterling games. In fact, we would talk about what time to go, and Dean would say that if we got into trouble, not to call him. Finally, he started going with us, and that was an ordeal. He got so mad and said not very nice things; then when he would leave to have a smoke, Linda and I would move to another seat and hope he wouldn't find us, but he always did.

Since we saw the students five days a week, we got to know them and knew they could come to us. For instance, there was a football player, and he was limping badly after a game. We asked him if he got hurt; he said his big toe hurt real bad. A couple days later, Linda noticed he was still limping but didn't look good, and he had a temperature. I was the first one off and took him to the school nurse; she got an appointment for him at the doctor's office. They started him on some powerful antibiotics and crutches. They said if it wasn't any better in four days, bring him back. We noticed one day that he wasn't in for lunch, and I knew where he lived. He was really sick, and I took him to the ER. The infection had gone systemic. He was in the hospital for a while, and his mother came from Colorado to take care of him. Linda and I would visit, and one day we ran into my daughter, Angie, and her friends. He couldn't believe that Angie was my daughter; they were classmates, and he was friends with Angie's boyfriend. He introduced his mother to us as the campus mothers. If my daughter were away at college, I would hope that a person like Linda was there to help.

Linda and I adopted two young men from Houston. I knew where they lived since Jennifer and Howard were living there. They were very nice, and they still say "yes, ma'am," and "no, ma'am." They always treated us with respect. We would always give them a hug before they would play ball. Their names are Roderick and Raymond Johnston, not related. Raymond was the football player, and his position was running back. Linda and I always traveled unless it was several hours away. At the end of the season, we would buy the little gold and blue football; then we would get his statistics from the year and mark it on the ball. He made a touchdown, and after the game, we were told that the touchdown that won the game, and while in the huddle, he wanted the ball and the touchdown for his moms.

Roderick played basketball, and we were there for

him. He was so excited to have us meet his parents. When we visited Jennifer and Howard, they asked us over for lunch at their home, and I got a big hug from Roderick. We really enjoyed their company, and Jennifer thought that was so nice and laughed at the way he and I looked at each other. During his sophomore year, he kind of got lost with life, but we got him back on the road. We talked about it at his house, and I told him that this year something special was going to happen. The team went all the way to the NAIA Championship but lost in the final game. I would call him before the game, and then Linda and I would listen to it on the radio. I kept all the newspaper write-ups, and he did well. I gave them to his parents.

Those boys each had special times with us. If they got sick, Linda would bake stuff for them and we would deliver it to their rooms.

They gave us memories, and when they graduated from college, it was hard to cut the umbilical cord, and it hurt to say good-bye. We decided that the kids knew to come to us for help, but we weren't going to get as close.

Linda and I continued having fun. But trouble would always be around the corner, it seemed.

Linda called late one night and asked if I wanted to ride with her to take a VHS tape back and pick up her son. It was in July and had been very hot and humid. We noticed how the heat was rising from the pavement on the highway and made it look like fog. Then, off in a distance, there was lightning in the clouds, and this set the stage.

Linda had noticed something strange in the ditch

while driving to McPherson, a fifteen-minute drive, at eleven thirty, and the tape had to be back by midnight or it was late. We got there in time, and then we went to pick her son up. Everyone seemed to be watering their yards that evening, and she thought it was funny to drive close to the curb and roll my window down so I would get wet. I was soaked by the time we were headed home. When we got to that place, she wanted to slow down and look to see what it was. We were all looking when we saw it was a body of a man. She turned around and rolled my window down so I could get a better look. It scared me to death; then her son had the bright idea of poking the man with a stick. We said no; he looked like someone had thrown him out like a rag doll. We weren't thinking to straight, and by the time we got to the city limits, Linda called 911 and explained where he was and that he had on a red and white checkered shirt. She asked if the sheriff wanted to meet us out there, and they said absolutely not and thanked us for the report. The next day, I heard that he had been a transient and had heatstroke. We felt good about calling it in, but did it have to be so spooky?

The summer before September 11, our families went to Disney World in Orlando for a week, and Howard and Jennifer met us at the airport to join us. Our departure at the airport in Kansas City was early, and we got an overnight room by the airport, and they took care of our cars. Linda wasn't sure about flying, so we asked her PA about it. She ordered two pills to take before boarding the plane.

While at the hotel, the men were in the bar, and we decided to go swimming. Linda's daughter, Kate, went with us. We decided to go sit in the hot tub, which was down in the gym. I didn't think that was too relaxing for some reason. Linda and I couldn't keep our bottoms on the seat and floated to the top, and that had to be no easy feat.

We started back to our rooms, and the door to the outside was locked, so we took the elevator but didn't know that our next stop was at a wedding reception. Here the three of us were, wet, hair a mess, beach towels wrapped around us, and no shoes. The door opened up, right at the reception, and of course people were watching the guests coming off the elevator. How embarrassing. We turned around and decided which way to escape because we already had been seen. We got out of there and hoped nobody recorded our entrance for *America's Funniest Home Videos.* They would have won the ten thousand dollars and the hundred thousand dollar pot. This was another fine mess we got ourselves into.

Linda had flown before, but it had been awhile. She had a couple Xanax and was told to take one while we were waiting to board the plane. Once on the plane, Tim, Linda's husband, and their daughters sat together, and Linda sat across the aisle from us in case she needed anything. She knew I was close but couldn't have cared less. We got her comfortable with a pillow and blanket; she was out before the plane took off and stayed out for three and a half hours. We got snacks, and Dean started to throw all his wrappers on her, and everybody followed. She sure was surprised when we woke her up, and we led her off the plane, but once we got walking through the airport, she came out of la-la land. It's still good for a laugh.

Our friendship hasn't always been perfect, especially when my anxiety came on, and I was mad at everybody and I couldn't figure out what was going on until I got medical help, but our friendship survived. Most of the problems were my fault, and I was really sorry for that. Linda once brought me a stuffed cow, and I named it LC for her initials; then we got to laughing about the Borden products and the cow on the commercial, but LC goes with me everywhere and helps my neck.

The last story about us is the best, and I'm sure glad I made Linda's day. We were having a real bad snowstorm, and we were asked to come in and help with dinner, and Linda said she would pick me up. Nobody could get to work who lived outside the town. She pulled up, and I very carefully came out and around the car to get in when she said I disappeared. One minute I was there; the next minute I was gone.

All of a sudden, I stood up, and I was packed with snow. I couldn't see, my glasses were full of snow, and my hair was soaked and cold. I was especially glad when she didn't have to potty because as hard as she laughed, the inside would have been wet too. We got to work, and she was still laughing and couldn't tell anyone what had happened; she'd start laughing all over again. She finally got a hold of herself until she drove back in the driveway, and you could see the area where I went down. It was a good thing it was fluffy. She still to this day cracks up about that snowy evening.

Unfortunately, we haven't been able to get together and go and do stuff, and since Dean and I moved, it has really hurt the two of us.

I crocheted an afghan when I was sitting with Mom, and I remember that Mom would sometimes watch me. She thought the colors that I had put together were beautiful. I finished the gift shortly after Mom had died, and I brought it to Linda while at work. I told her that when she cuddles in the afghan to always think that my arms are around her, giving her a big hug. Thanks, Linda, for all the fun, laughter, and all those ridiculous times.

Dean told me to tell another story, so here we go. During the summer, Tim was gone on a business trip, and it was too hot to do anything at home, so she brought the cartoon, *Foghorn Leghorn,* about the sheepdog that watched over the sheep herd and the rooster on DVD. She brought over a bottle of wine, and the doctor told me that I could have wine once in awhile. So we drank it from straws that had eyeballs, and when you sipped through them, they looked at you. Anyway, the first bottle wasn't very big but tasted so good. I had one in the refrigerator, and we started on the next bottle. The cartoons got funnier, and everything was funny until she sat in the recliner and the bolt came out, and she thought that she had broke the chair, which she hadn't, so we tipped it over and started trying to get the bolt back, but it was hard to hit the hole. Dean came walking in the door and found both of our heads in the chair and our bottoms up in the air. He couldn't believe the shape we were in and in the middle of the afternoon. He even yelled at us, but that was useless; we just kept laughing at each other. It ended up that Angie and her friend got Linda home; Angie drove her car, and the friend followed. Dean gave me two aspirins and an ice pack. He thought that I would need it pretty soon.

A couple days later, I had an appointment with my doctor, and Dean tattled on me. He asked if it was okay for me to drink wine, and the doctor didn't think it would hurt me once in awhile. Dean then asked what about sharing two bottles, and he told me that I didn't do a real smart thing. He meant two to three ounces at a time. All's well that ends well.

THE CONCLUSION OF THE FAMILY PRESCRIPTION: A HISTORY OF A FAMILY

There Are No Simple Answers

Some of the problems start in the home and some elsewhere. Where do we start?

First of all, stop pointing fingers at each other; we probably all are at blame. Where is the responsibility in our daily life? On the Internet, I found the NIDA (National Institute On Drug Abuse) and a letter written by Nora D. Volkow M.D., the director. The last paragraph says:

> I want to remind young people, their parents, and others that even though prescription drugs

are medications, their improper use can have serious consequences. I'd encourage parents, their parents, and other adults to check out their medicine cabinets and to discard any prescription drugs that are no longer required to treat a medical condition so that these medications are not available to be misused.

Physicians and Pharmacists

I have noticed that the physicians and pharmacies are trying new ways of watching and accounting for all the medications that are passed out. I have seen my doctor doing things a little different. I need to take prescriptions because if I didn't, I probably wouldn't be alive. But if my grandson would take what I take every day, well, I'm afraid of what might happen.

We have to remember that these people who have studied so hard still take classes and tests to refine their abilities. They are human beings, not God. They make mistakes, and some mistakes stay around the rest of my life. Have you forgotten what happened to me? No! There was no sense of it; wrong is wrong. I did not sue. I have just toughed it out, and my anger is still there, especially when something does go wrong.

Heroes, Very Few and Far Between

Who do our children have to look up to anymore? Actors, sports personalities (college and professionals), or anyone who is nationally known. There is a responsibility that you provide, even if you don't think there is. Children and young adults are watching what you have done to your bodies to get ahead in this life. Teachers, coaches, politicians, even parents and grandparents are being watched. Our young adults are trying to be like their heroes. Let's show them how they should live their lives by cleaning our messes up or staying out of the limelight.

The Internet

The Internet is a fantastic form of knowledge. I feel my generation was really cheated. But there is the old saying about how one bad apple can spoil a bushel basket. I have been investigating about the abuse of steroids, since I'm interested in this problem, and all the different sites where anyone can buy legal steroids. This still causes problems. Since it is on the Internet, everything is up for grabs, legal or not. Let's help our newest generation clean up.

Life and the Future

With the problems with my endocrine system, taking the steroids, and now with type 2 diabetes, they fight against each other, plus the problem with anxiety, I never know what tomorrow will bring. I guess no one does. I have had many surgeries to repair my feet because of the steroids but have managed to finally have them fixed.

I tackled another problem last summer. I had not seen a movie at the theater in almost seven years. I have really never figured out the problem, whether it's the sound systems or the lights; it's anyone's guess. But Dean and I went to the drive-in theater and watched a new movie. I felt that this was the movie to see and had the windows open for lots of fresh air. I didn't leave the car for anything; I stayed strapped in my seatbelt and really enjoyed the movie. Jennifer and family were right next to us, and I felt that I had accomplished a lot. Sometimes anxiety, for no reason, shows its nasty side, and I try to control it with breathing and some other relaxation methods and even with feedback. But I have medication if I can't manage it, only if I can't control the feeling. Writing this book has done wonders for me, and I always find someone worse off than me. I also keep a diary; I write whatever I want. There is an understanding with Dean that if something were to happen to me, no one will ever read it, and it will be burned. I've been writing for more than three years. This has helped with the hormone imbalance of the chemical serotonin that causes the anxiety. I have had to study a lot to learn about my body, and looking back, I would have gone through the withdrawal and everything else.

Well, this has been my story and I am pretty sure there is more to come, but I still worry about the kids today. I think that there is a different way to advertise the problem. The commercials that are out now, just don't do it and the one that says" just say no!" Forget it. Maybe by reading the book, you can do some research yourself on the internet. You could even come up with your own idea.

Remember to always tell your children you love them or show them by holding or just by putting your hand on their shoulder. All it takes is that one, four letter word—LOVE. You just never know. You also hope that you have talked to them or at least they will remember about the do's and don'ts. It only takes a minute and their gone.

In my Introduction, I asked the questions about using somebody else's medication or lending some of your medication to someone else. I have to admit it, I have done this before. Shame on me!